FELINE AND CANINE INFECTIOUS DISEASES

LIBRARY OF VETERINARY PRACTICE

FELINE AND CANINE INFECTIOUS DISEASES

ROSALIND M. GASKELL BVSc, PhD, MRCVS
Reader, Faculty of Veterinary Science, University of Liverpool

and

MALCOLM BENNETT BVSc, PhD, MRCVS
Lecturer, Faculty of Veterinary Science, University of Liverpool

with

BRYN TENNANT BVSc, PhD, Cert VR, MRCVS
VIO, SAC Veterinary Services, Penicuik

and

KIM WILLOUGHBY BVMS, MRCVS
Feline Advisory Bureau Scholar, Faculty of Veterinary Science, University of Liverpool

Blackwell
Science

© 1996 by
Blackwell Science Ltd
Editorial Offices:
Osney Mead, Oxford OX2 0EL
25 John Street, London WC1N 2BL
23 Ainslie Place, Edinburgh EH3 6AJ
238 Main Street, Cambridge,
   Massachusetts 02142, USA
54 University Street, Carlton,
   Victoria 3053, Australia

Other Editorial Offices:
Arnette Blackwell SA
   224, Boulevard Saint Germain
   75007 Paris, France

Blackwell Wissenschafts-Verlag GmbH
   Kurfürstendamm 57
   10707 Berlin, Germany

   Zehetnergasse 6
   A-1140 Wien, Austria

First published 1996

Set in 10/12 Souvenir
by DP Photosetting, Aylesbury, Bucks
Printed and bound in Great Britain
by Hartnolls Ltd., Bodmin, Cornwall

DISTRIBUTORS

Marston Book Services Ltd
PO Box 87
Oxford OX2 0DT
(Orders: Tel: 01865 791155
         Fax: 01865 791927
         Telex: 837515)

USA
Blackwell Science, Inc.
238 Main Street
Cambridge, MA 02142
(Orders: Tel: 800 215-1000
              617 876-7000
         Fax: 617 492-5263)

Canada
Copp Clark, Ltd
2775 Matheson Blvd East
Mississauga, Ontario
Canada, L4W 4P7
(Orders: Tel: 800 263-4374
              905 238-6074)

Australia
Blackwell Science Pty Ltd
54 University Street,
Carlton, Victoria 3053
(Orders: Tel: 03 9347-0300
         Fax: 03 9349-3016)

A catalogue record for this title
is available from the British Library

ISBN 0–632–03446–7

Library of Congress
Cataloging in Publication Data
is available

LIBRARY OF VETERINARY PRACTICE

Editors

J.B. Sutton, *JP, MRCVS*
S.T. Swift, *MA, VetMB, CertSAC, MRCVS*

CONTENTS

PREFACE

This book was conceived as a result of many years of producing course notes both for veterinary undergraduates and for continuing education meetings aimed at veterinary practitioners and interested dog and cat owners. Because the book originated as lecture notes, we hope that the information it contains will be reasonably comprehensive, but that the format will make it readily accessible and digestible. We intend that the book should be used for easy reference to basic information about a disease; for updating of current knowledge; and for revision purposes if you are in the unfortunate position of having to pass an exam. However, we hope the book will be user-friendly enough to browse through at any time and for any motive.

Small animal infectious diseases range from the fast moving feline retrovirus field, with feline leukaemia and feline immunodeficiency virus infections, to diseases such as feline panleucopenia where our practical knowledge and advice has changed little in over twenty years. We have also included some newly recognised infections and some more exotic ones which we hope the reader will find stimulating. Although the book is not referenced as such, for those of more academic bent there is a list of several fully referenced texts provided at the back, and some selected recent and topical references are also given to tempt your interest.

We would welcome feedback from readers regarding any errors of both omission or fact that may inadvertently be present, and would also welcome suggestions as to how the book's usefulness may be improved in the future.

LIST OF ABBREVIATIONS

AZT	3′-Azido-3′deoxythymidine
BSE	Bovine spongiform encephalopathy
CAV	Canine adenovirus
CCV	Canine coronavirus
CDV	Canine distemper virus
CHV	Canine herpesvirus
CMI	Cell-mediated immunity
CNS	Central nervous system
CPV	Canine parvovirus
CPIV	Canine parainfluenza virus
CRV	Canine rotavirus
CSD	Cat scratch disease
ELISA	Enzyme-linked immunosorbent assay
FCV	Feline calicivirus
FECV	Feline enteric coronavirus
FCoV	Feline coronavirus
FeLV	Feline leukaemia virus
FeSFV	Feline syncitium-forming virus
FeSV	Feline sarcoma virus
FHV	Feline herpesvirus
FIPV	Feline infectious peritonitis virus
FIV	Feline immunodeficiency virus
FP	Feline panleucopenia
FSE	Feline spongiform encephalopathy
FUS	Feline urological syndrome
HI	Haemagglutination-inhibiting
ICH	Infectious canine hepatitis
IF	Immunofluorescence
Ig	Immunoglobulin
IM	Intramuscular
IV	Intravenous
LCMV	Lymphochoriomeningitis virus
MDA	Maternally derived antibody
MHCII	Major histocompatibility complex type II

PCR	Polymerase chain reaction
RIPA	Radioimmune precipitation assays
RMSF	Rocky Mountain spotted fever
SAF	Scrapie associated fibrils
SC	Subcutaneous
SPD	Salmon poisoning disease
URD	Upper respiratory disease
VN	Virus neutralising

Section 1
MAJOR FELINE
INFECTIOUS DISEASES

1   FELINE INFECTIOUS RESPIRATORY DISEASE

This chapter is divided into four parts:

(1) **Viral respiratory disease**. The majority of cases of infectious respiratory disease in cats are caused by one of two viruses, feline calicivirus (FCV) or feline herpesvirus (FHV) (feline rhinotracheitis virus).

(2) **Feline *Chlamydia psittaci* infection**. This organism mainly induces conjunctivitis, though mild respiratory signs may also be present.

(3) ***Bordetella bronchiseptica* infection**. *B. bronchiseptica* is undoubtedly important in secondary infections, but recently evidence has been accumulating that it may also be important as a primary pathogen in cats.

(4) **Mycoplasma infection**. Again these are most likely to be important as secondary invaders, but a more primary role has been suggested by some.

Other viruses with only suspected or peripheral involvement include feline reovirus (*see* Chapter 20), cowpox virus (Chapter 6) and feline coronavirus (Chapter 3).

Other bacteria such as staphylococci, streptococci, pasteurellae and coliforms are also important as secondary invaders.

VIRAL RESPIRATORY DISEASE

AETIOLOGY

Feline herpesvirus (FHV)

- An alphaherpesvirus, containing double-stranded DNA, with a glycoprotein–lipid envelope.
- Only one serotype; isolates also very similar on restriction enzyme analysis of DNA.
- Most isolates are of similar, uniform pathogenicity, though attenuated vaccine strains do exist and, in contrast, some strains appear to induce more severe disease.

- Comparatively labile in the external environment (survives up to approximately 24 hours depending on temperature and relative humidity).
- Envelope makes it susceptible to all common disinfectants, e.g. hypochlorite, quaternary ammonium compounds.
- Only appears to infect members of the cat family; isolates have been obtained from dogs but the significance of this is unclear.

Feline calicivirus (FCV)

- Small unenveloped single-stranded RNA virus.
- Cup-like depressions on surface from which 'calicivirus' name derived.
- One main serotype but antigenic variation within this.
- Although most strains are closely related, there are some differences in pathogenicity and in the degree of cross-protection between strains.
- Survives for up to approximately 1 week in external environment, depending on temperature and relative humidity.
- Susceptible to low pH but not all disinfectants: hypochlorite and quaternary ammonium compounds satisfactory.
- Only appears to infect members of the cat family, although caliciviruses antigenically similar to FCV have been recovered from dogs.

PATHOGENESIS AND PATHOLOGY

Feline herpesvirus infection

The natural route of infection is intranasal, oral or conjunctival, though experimentally other routes have been investigated. Inoculation of pregnant queens by the vaginal route has led to vaginitis and congenitally infected kittens, and intravenous inoculation has led to transplacental infection and abortion. A predilection of the virus for the growth regions of the skeleton, including the turbinates, has been shown following intravenous inoculation of young kittens.

In the typical respiratory infection, however, virus replication takes place predominantly in the mucosae of the nasal septum, turbinates, nasopharynx and tonsils; other tissues including conjunctivae, mandibular lymph nodes and upper trachea are also often involved. Virus may be detected in secretions 24 hours after inoculation and persists for 1–3 weeks. Viraemia has only rarely been detected and virus replication in visceral tissues is uncommon.

Pathological findings

These may be summarised as follows:

Gross:

- Most significant lesions of focal necrosis and mucoid to mucopurulent exudate present in upper respiratory tract, particularly nasal passages and turbinates.

- Milder areas of inflammation may be present elsewhere, e.g. trachea, conjunctivae.

Histopathology:

- Virus replication in epithelium shown by presence of intranuclear inclusion bodies.
- Areas of multifocal epithelial degeneration and necrosis.
- Predominantly neutrophil infiltration and exudation with fibrin.

Resolution:

- Epithelial regeneration with some squamous cell metaplasia, and sometimes hypertrophy, over 2–3 weeks.

Feline calicivirus infection

The natural routes of infection are also intranasal, oral or conjunctival. There are differences between some strains in their tissue tropisms and pathogenicity. For the typical oral or respiratory isolate, virus replication takes place mainly in the tissues of the oral cavity, upper respiratory tract and conjunctivae. Some strains also appear to have a predilection for joints, and some for the lungs. However, lung involvement may have been overemphasised in the past owing to the use of aerosols in some experimental studies, rather than the more natural intranasal route. Virus may also sometimes be found in visceral tissues, faeces and, occasionally, urine.

Pathological findings

Thus pathological findings vary according to the strain:

- Ulcers on the dorsal surface of the tongue are usually a prominent feature.
- Ulcers may also occur elsewhere, for example on the hard palate, lips and external nares.
- Changes in upper respiratory and conjunctival epithelium less marked.
- Ulcers begin as vesicles which subsequently rupture with necrosis of the overlying epithelium and infiltration by neutrophils at the periphery and base.
- Virus replication in joints appears to be in synovial macrophages, with gross and histopathological findings of acute synovitis.
- Pulmonary lesions result from initial focal alveolitis, which leads to areas of acute exudative pneumonia and finally a proliferative interstitial pneumonia.

CLINICAL SIGNS

Feline herpesvirus infection

This generally causes a severe upper respiratory disease particularly in young, susceptible animals. The incubation period is usually 2–6 days, but may be longer. A higher infecting dose can lead to a shorter incubation period and more severe clinical signs.

The following features may be seen:

- Early signs of depression, marked sneezing, inappetance, pyrexia and sometimes hypersalivation.
- As the disease progresses, marked ocular and nasal discharges develop; also conjunctivitis, and sometimes dyspnoea and coughing.
- A leucocytosis with left shift is present.
- More rarely, ulcerative or interstitial keratitis may occur.
- Occasionally tongue ulcers may be seen, but these are much less common than in FCV infection.
- Other signs seen rarely include skin ulcers, primary viral pneumonia, and nervous signs.
- Occasionally generalised disease seen in young or immunosuppressed animals.
- Abortion may occur but only as a result of severe debilitating disease and not the direct effect of virus itself.
- The mortality rate is not usually high except sometimes in young kittens. Fatalities most often result from dehydration and secondary bacterial infection which may lead to bronchopneumonia.
- Resolution is usually within 2–3 weeks, although severe necrosis of mucous membranes, particularly turbinates, may lead to chronic rhinitis and sinusitis.
- Persistent/recurrent signs may also follow recurrent virus shedding from carriers.

Feline calicivirus infection

FCV infection is typically milder than FHV, although there are different strains of feline calicivirus which can cause a spectrum of disease ranging from a relatively severe syndrome through to a subclinical infection.

However, certain features of FCV infection may be used to help differentiate it from FHV infection.

- Usually much milder with little general malaise.
- Transient pyrexia; only mild sneezing and conjunctivitis present.
- Ocular and nasal discharges less prominent.
- Mouth ulceration is a frequent and characteristic feature and may occur as the only clinical sign.

- Ulcers may occur on tongue, soft and hard palate, lips, and median cleft of nostrils.
- Inflammation of the fauces may be present – this may be relevant to the development of chronic lesions in this site (see below).
- No keratitis or hypersalivation, although some cats with severe ulcers may show slight wetness around the mouth.
- Some strains cause pyrexia and lameness, which may or may not be accompanied by oral or respiratory signs.
- Some strains produce an interstitial pneumonia; dyspnoea may be the main feature.
- Diarrhoea may occasionally occur.

FCV may play a role in chronic oral lesions in cats: some studies have shown that a higher proportion of cats with this syndrome are FCV carriers compared with unaffected control cats. However, this condition is also associated with feline immunodeficiency virus (FIV) infection (see Chapter 5).

There is some evidence that concurrent FIV infection may potentiate FCV infection. This may partly explain the apparent association of these two viruses in the field in cases of chronic stomatitis, but the pathogenesis of the syndrome is still unclear.

DIAGNOSIS

To a large extent the diseases caused by the two viruses may be distinguished on the presenting clinical signs. Table 1.1 summarises the main features of each condition and also includes feline *Chlamydia psittaci* and *Bordetella bronchiseptica* infection (pages 21 and 25) as a differential diagnosis.

A number of factors can influence the outcome of infection and can make it more difficult to distinguish the cause of the disease.

There may be differences in virulence between virus strains and also the level of the infecting virus dose can affect the severity of the disease seen. The cat itself can influence the response, for example, with factors such as:

- age;
- genotype;
- general health;
- nutritional status;
- intercurrent disease (e.g. with feline leukaemia virus (FeLV), FIV, feline panleucopenia);
- differences in microbial flora (more severe syndromes may be associated with beta-haemolytic streptococci, haemolytic staphylococci, *Pasteurella multocida*, and *B. bronchiseptica* infection);
- specific immune status, i.e. the cat may be partially or wholly immune from vaccination or a previous infection, or a kitten may have maternally derived antibody.

Table 1.1 A comparison of the essential features of respiratory infections in cats

	FHV	FCV*	FCh†	Bb^tt
general malaise	+++	+	+	+
sneezing	+++	+	+	++
conjunctivitis	++	++	+++**	−
hypersalivation	++	−^	−	−
ocular discharge	+++	++	+++	(+)
nasal discharge	+++	++	+	++
oral ulceration	+	+++	−	−
keratitis	+	−	−	−
coughing	(+)	−	−	++
pneumonia	(+)	+	+/−	+
lameness	−	++	−	−

* strain variation
** often·persistent
(+) uncommon, but may occur
+/− lesions may be present, but not usually seen clinically
−^ slight wetness may be seen around the mouth if ulcers present

†FCh = *Chlamydia psittaci* infection
tt Bb = *Bordetella bronchiseptica* infection

Confirming diagnosis

Diagnosis may be confirmed by isolation of the agent. Oropharyngeal swabs should be placed immediately in viral transport media and sent by first class post to a specialist laboratory, preferably at the beginning of the week. If this is not possible, short-term (less than 1 day) storage at 4°C, or longer term (less than 2 weeks) at −20°C should be satisfactory.

Samples should be taken ideally within one week of the onset of clinical signs. If chlamydial infection is suspected, a firmly taken conjunctival swab should be sent in chlamydial transport medium to a specialist laboratory. In unvaccinated cats serology may be helpful in establishing a diagnosis of chlamydial infection (Part 2 of this chapter).

Interpreting results

When virus is successfully isolated from a case of acute respiratory disease, it is reasonable to assume that in most cases it is the actual cause. However, one or more pathogens may be involved in any one case, and also, particularly for feline calicivirus, the results may be equivocal because of the large proportion of apparently healthy cats that also carry, and actively shed, the virus (see 'Epidemiology').

Bacterial culture and sensitivity tests

Bacterial culture and sensitivity testing is important in cases where discharges are copious and purulent and which fail to respond to an initial course of antibiotics.

The most valuable material is obtained from the nasal chambers, after the nares have been cleaned with antiseptic solution.

TREATMENT

Acute upper respiratory disease

Antiviral drugs

Although several anti-herpesvirus drugs have been used successfully in other species, none is in common usage for FHV. However, for ulcerative keratitis due to FHV, a 0.1% ophthalmic solution of 5-iododeoxyuridine 4–6 times daily for 3–5 days has been recommended although not licensed for cats. Acyclovir, commonly used for herpes simplex virus infection in man, does not appear to have as much activity against FHV, at least *in vitro*.

Antibiotics

A broad-spectrum antibiotic (e.g. ampicillin, potentiated sulphonamide or oxytetracycline) to control secondary bacterial infection should be used. Paediatric syrups or long-acting injections may be useful if swallowing is painful. If *B. bronchiseptica* or *C. psittaci* involvement is suspected, then doxycycline or oxytetracycline is indicated. Cats should be re-examined after 4–5 days, and antibiotics continued if necessary. If there is no improvement after a week, bacterial culture and sensitivity tests should be carried out.

Supportive vitamin care

Vitamins A, B and C as oral drops; and vitamin B_{12} may be helpful.

Corticosteroids

These are contraindicated as they retard the healing process and may potentiate the virus infection.

Fluid therapy

In mild cases of dehydration, food liquidised with added water may be adequate. In more severe cases subcutaneous or intravenous fluid therapy may be necessary, bearing in mind that, where dehydration is severe, fluid may not be adequately absorbed by the subcutaneous route. In prolonged cases of anorexia and dehydration, a gastrotomy tube might be indicated.

Nursing

This is often best done at home by the owner as cats do respond positively to attention. Purring can also help clear the airways! Hospital intensive care requires scrupulous hygiene to prevent cross-infection. Affected cats should be kept in a clean, warm, well ventilated environment, and kept groomed. Discharges should be wiped away and a bland ointment applied to prevent excoriation.

Feeding

Aromatic and strongly flavoured foods (e.g. sardines, pilchards) should be offered. If oral ulceration makes eating painful, baby foods or specialised proprietary or liquidised food should be given.

Nebulisers and steam inhalation

Nebulisers and steam inhalation (e.g. sitting the cat in a steamy bathroom) to clear airways are tolerated better by cats than are nasal decongestants.

Chronic upper respiratory disease

Prevention

Ideally there should be adequate therapy for secondary bacterial infection in the acute stage of the disease. Once the intranasal structures are irreversibly damaged, the long term prognosis is relatively poor.

Bacterial culture and sensitivity tests

Bacterial culture and sensitivity tests can be performed and cats treated for at least 3 weeks. Chronic rhinitis classically improves after a prolonged course of antibiotics, although often only temporarily. If no improvement is seen, then concurrent infection with FIV or FeLV or other, much rarer diagnoses such as nasal mycoses or neoplasia should be considered.

Mucolytics

Mucolytics, e.g. bromhexine hydrochloride, may be useful.

Local infusion of antibiotics

This may help, but often seems to have no real advantage in the chronic phase over the oral and parenteral routes.

Surgery

Radical surgical excision of diseased tissues has been advocated, but the surgery itself is poorly tolerated by cats.

Housing

Sometimes cats improve on being kept predominantly outdoors.

Prognosis

Long-term prognosis is, unfortunately, poor.

EPIDEMIOLOGY

Both FHV and FCV are highly successful pathogens of the cat and, despite vaccination, infection and disease still occur. The viruses are generally less common in isolated household pets than in colony animals. Thus the disease occurs mainly in boarding catteries, breeding colonies, stray cat homes, or other situations where a large number of cats have been brought together.

The feline respiratory viruses persist in such populations in three main ways:

- By passing directly from acutely infected to susceptible animals: this depends on sufficient numbers of susceptible animals in the population, and sufficient opportunities for contact between them.
- By persisting in the environment: although this is for only relatively short periods of time, it is long enough for indirect transmission to occur, particularly within the close confines of a cattery via contaminated secretions on cages, feeding bowls, cleaning utensils or personnel.
- By persisting in the recovered cat by means of carriers.

There are no known reservoirs or alternative hosts for these viruses, and *in utero* transmission does not generally seem to occur.

With both viruses the carrier state is a common phenomenon, and probably the main reason why these viruses are so successful.

Features of the FHV carrier state (Figure 1.1)

- The carrier state is characterised by latency (i.e. no infectious virus detectable in oronasal and conjunctival secretions) with intermittent episodes of detectable virus shedding.
- At least 80% of recovered cats remain as viral carriers.
- Approximately half of these are likely to be of epidemiological importance (likely to shed virus under natural conditions).
- Shedding may occur spontaneously, but is most likely after a stress, e.g. corticosteroid treatment, a change of housing such as going into a boarding cattery, to a cat show or to stud, and kittening and lactation.
- Shedding does not occur immediately after the stress; there is a lag period of about 1 week, followed by a shedding episode of from 1 to 2 weeks.

Thus the total probable infectious period after a stress is about 3 weeks.

- Carrier animals may show mild clinical signs during the shedding episode.

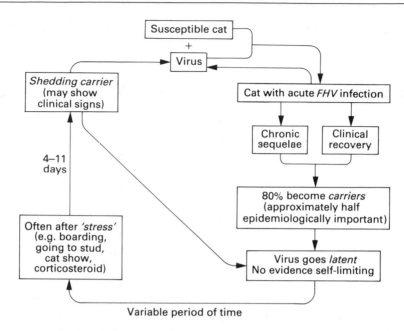

Figure 1.1 FHV 1 carrier state: epidemiology

- There is no evidence that the carrier state is self limiting, although there is some evidence of a refractory period for a few months after an episode of shedding during which animals are less likely to shed virus again.
- As with some other herpesvirus infections, the virus remains latent in trigeminal ganglia but recent evidence has shown that other tissues may also be involved.

Practical implications of these findings

- FHV carriers are difficult to identify because they only shed virus intermittently. Virus shedding is more likely to occur after a stress, but this cannot be relied upon.
- In an infected colony, most cats will be carriers, although some individuals may be more likely to shed than others. For example, some queens may repeatedly produce infected litters and it may be advisable to use other queens for breeding.
- Any individual animal with a history of respiratory disease, or with persistent or recurrent signs, is likely to be a carrier.
- FHV carriers should always be regarded as potentially infectious as they may shed virus spontaneously at any time. However, they are likely to be particularly dangerous in the 3-week period after they have undergone any stress (see above).
- A recurrence of mild clinical signs may indicate the cat is actually shedding virus.
- Vaccinated cats may be carriers because they were infected either before vaccination or after. They may never have shown clinical signs.

- Kittens may become carriers under protection of maternally derived antibody and again may not have shown clinical signs.

Features of the FCV carrier state (Figure 1.2)

- Unlike FHV, FCV carriers shed virus more or less continuously, and are therefore always infectious to other cats.
- In some cats the carrier state is lifelong, but most animals at some point spontaneously recover and appear to eliminate virus.
- In experimental studies where carriers have been produced, most cats were still shedding FCV 30 days after infection. By 75 days, 50% were shedding. The proportion shedding continues to decline, although some animals become long-term carriers. In other studies, the carrier state has been difficult to reproduce, suggesting that there may be virus strain differences or, perhaps, host or other factors that may play a role.
- There is some evidence that pre-existing FIV infection may increase the proportion of cats that become FCV carriers, and the length of time they shed.
- Carriers may be divided arbitrarily into three groups – high-, medium- and low-level excretors, each shedding a fairly constant amount of virus which fluctuates around a mean for that individual cat. High-level excretors are highly infectious and easily detected on swabbing; low-level excretors are less infectious and a series of swabs may be necessary to identify them.
- Feline calicivirus carriers are very widespread: surveys show that approximately 20% of cats attending a veterinary hospital and general practice for reasons other than oral/respiratory disease were FCV carriers, and 25% of apparently healthy cats at cat shows. These figures are very similar to those obtained in surveys carried out over 20 years ago before vaccination when

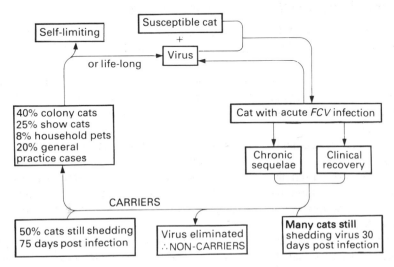

Figure 1.2 FCV carrier state: epidemiology

approximately 40% of cats in colonies, 25% of show cats and 8% of household pets were positive.

- Virus persists in tonsil and other oropharyngeal tissues, but unfortunately tonsillectomy does not cure carriers.

Practical implications of these findings

FCV carriers may be identified by isolation of virus from a single oropharyngeal swab, although several samples over a 4- to 6-week period are preferable. Since cats can eliminate virus at any point, it is worth retesting at a later date if required. A positive swab usually indicates the cat is a carrier, but it may be undergoing transient reinfection, or it may be infected with a non-pathogenic strain. Cats can become vaccine virus carriers after use of intranasal vaccine.

Where virus isolation is not carried out, potential carriers may be identified on clinical history and circumstantial evidence, as for FHV carriers.

Vaccinated animals may also be field virus carriers, and kittens may become carriers under cover of maternally derived antibody, as for FHV.

Summary

Viral respiratory disease appears wherever cats are congregated together, and the viruses are often introduced by the clinically normal carrier. The pattern of enzootic viral respiratory disease in such a colony is shown in Figure 1.3.

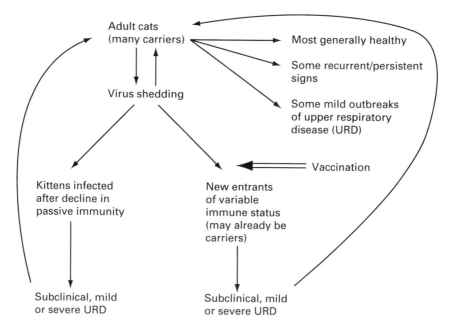

Figure 1.3 Pattern of enzootic viral respiratory disease in a colony

TRANSMISSION

- Transmission is mainly through direct cat-to-cat contact through infectious discharges – oral, nasal and conjunctival secretions. For FCV, virus may also be in urine and faeces, although probably not important epidemiologically.
- Indirect transmission may occur in the short-term, particularly in catteries. Contaminated secretions may be present on cages, personnel, and feeding and cleaning utensils. Not of long-term significance since viruses relatively short-lived outside the cat.
- Aerosol transmission is not thought to be of major significance though sneezed macrodroplets may travel over 1–2 m.
- Transmission is reduced where measures are taken to minimise external virus survival, e.g. disinfection, optimum environmental temperature, low relative humidity, and adequate ventilation (15–20 air changes an hour).
- Efficacy of transmission depends on amount of virus being shed by infecting animal, and duration and intimacy of contact. Although the concentration of virus in the secretions of carriers and acutely infected cats may be similar, the viruses spread more easily from acute cases, probably because discharges are more copious. However, carriers are undoubtedly important, particularly with the close contact seen in colonies.

IMMUNITY

For both viruses this has generally been measured by serum virus neutralising (VN) antibody titres, though for FHV particularly, other immune mechanisms, especially cellular immunity, may be a truer reflection of immune status. Even for FCV, where VN antibody was traditionally considered to be the hallmark of immunity, some cats with no detectable VN antibody may show immunity to rechallenge with a heterologous FCV strain. The ultimate test of immunity is, of course, response to challenge.

In FHV, just after initial infection, cats are generally resistant to challenge, although VN antibody titres are generally low and in some cases undetectable. After six months or more, however, protection may only be partial and indeed carrier cats may reinfect themselves at any time. Following exogenous or endogenous reinfection, VN antibody titres rise to more moderate levels and thereafter, independent of virus shedding episodes, remain relatively stable.

In FCV, VN antibody titres are higher than those in FHV, and immunity following natural infection is thought to be longer lived. However, there is some variation depending on the virus strain involved and whether or not homotypic or heterotypic responses are being considered.

The duration of immunity following vaccination is not known. Most challenge studies have been done within 3 months of vaccination, but equivalent protection has been reported for FHV after a year and for FCV 10–12 months. Most manufacturers recommend yearly revaccination or 6-monthly in some circumstances.

Maternally derived antibody (essentially colostral) in kittens may persist for 2–10 weeks for FHV (mean levels falling below detectable (less than 1 in 2) levels by 9 weeks of age). For FCV, titres may be more persistent, antibody declining to undetectable levels by 10–14 weeks of age. However, for FCV, low levels of maternally derived antibody do not necessarily protect against infection or disease. In contrast, some kittens with no detectable FHV antibody appeared to be protected against disease, though not infection.

PREVENTION AND CONTROL

Vaccination has been available for a number of years, and has generally been successful in controlling the disease. However, disease still occurs in some colonies, particularly in young kittens as they lose their maternally derived antibody, and in open colonies such as stray cat homes. Both viruses are extremely widespread in the cat population and clinically healthy carriers are common, ensuring plenty of exposure. Thus prevention and control often require a combined approach of vaccination and management.

Vaccination

Three types of vaccine are available in the UK for the protection of cats against viral upper respiratory disease:

- Attenuated live vaccines given systemically.
- Attenuated live vaccine given intranasally.
- Inactivated, adjuvanted vaccines given systemically.

Table 1.2 gives the advantages and disadvantages of the different vaccines.

Genetically engineered strains of FHV have also been developed for use as vaccines.

Although the feline respiratory virus vaccines are, in general, reasonably effective, problems do occur from time to time. It has been suggested that most problems associated with feline respiratory virus vaccines are related to FCV rather than FHV, though both do occur.

Apparent vaccine reactions

(Defined as clinical disease which appears within a week or so of vaccination.)

Clinical signs commonly reported as vaccine reactions include upper respiratory and ocular signs, mouth ulceration, and in many cases also, lameness and fever. Typically such reactions occur approximately 6–7 days after vaccination, often after primary vaccination of young kittens, and it has been sug-

Table 1.2 Advantages and disadvantages of different vaccines

	Advantages	Disadvantages
Attenuated systemic	Several different ones available	Original FCV vaccines based on strain F9. Most vaccines protect against majority of isolates, but not as well against all
	Convenient to administer	Care needed with administration since if reaches oral/respiratory mucosa by mistake, can cause disease. Should not generalise, but can do in some cases
Intranasal	Induces better and more rapid (2–4 day) protection; useful for stray cat homes or during disease outbreak	More difficult to administer Side effects of sneezing and sometimes other signs may be seen
	May be useful in young kittens	
Inactivated systemic	Convenient to administer	Adjuvants may occasionally cause reaction
	Safe in pregnant queens	May not be such good immunity
	Useful in virus-free colonies	
	No reversion to virulence	

gested that this syndrome may be associated with the FCV component of particular vaccines. Whilst some of the isolates appear to be similar to vaccine virus, many of them appear to be field viruses.

Possible causes

- Cat already incubating the disease – vaccination programmes are usually implemented when kittens are highly susceptible to infection because of waning maternally derived antibody. Carriers are widespread and ensure that there is plenty of field virus around.
- Cat may already be a field virus carrier, and may show recurrent or persistent signs related to damage from the original infection. For FHV too, the mild stress and disruption of routine during vaccination may stimulate an episode of virus shedding in some carriers.
- Vaccine virus given by wrong route, i.e. attenuated live systemic vaccine inadvertently given by oronasal route as a result of aerosol from a syringe, or a cat licking the injection site of itself or others. In some cases even where the

vaccine has been given correctly, vaccine virus may generalise and reach the oropharynx.

- Intranasal vaccination quite often results in mild sneezing and occasional cases of ocular or nasal discharges and oral ulceration.
- Individual animals may be immunologically compromised through inter-current disease (e.g. FeLV, FIV, feline panleucopenia), or have particularly opportunist secondary microbial flora.

Apparent vaccine breakdowns

(When the cat was apparently successfully vaccinated but disease occurs within the normal recommended period of immunity.)

Possible causes

Assuming the vaccine was potent and had been stored and given correctly, other possible causes include the following:

- Although protection from the current vaccines is reasonable, even under ideal circumstances, protection is not necessarily complete in all cats.
- Intercurrent disease, e.g. with FeLV or FIV, either at the time of vaccination or thereafter. There is evidence from experimental studies that previous infection with FIV renders subsequent vaccination with an inactivated FCV vaccine significantly less effective in protecting against FCV challenge.
- Overwhelming infection. Studies have shown that the majority of vaccine breakdowns occur approximately 6 months after vaccination, and it may be that as immunity declines, a high challenge dose could overcome lowered levels.
- Maternally derived antibody may have interfered with initial vaccination programme. The duration of maternal immunity in kittens can be variable, and there is little information on the interaction between this and vaccination.
- Other agents not incorporated in the vaccine may be causing disease, e.g. feline *C. psittaci, B. bronchiseptica.*
- Although most vaccines incorporate strains of FCV that are reasonably cross-reactive (e.g. F9), they do not appear to protect equally well against all strains of FCV. The vaccines may therefore not provide complete protection against some of the viruses isolated from vaccine breakdowns. For the FHV component this is not such a problem, since there is only one antigenic strain, which seems relatively stable.
- Carriers: the common occurrence of carriers ensures there is a ready supply of virus to infect susceptible cats. Vaccination does not eliminate infection from cats that are already carriers, and a previously unexposed cat systemically vaccinated can become a field virus carrier if later exposed to field virus. Intranasally vaccinated cats may become carriers of the attenuated FCV vaccine component, but there is some evidence that intranasal vaccination may protect in the short term against cats becoming FHV field virus carriers.

Management measures

Different circumstances may require different approaches, as outlined below.

Household pets

These should be vaccinated routinely, and given a booster vaccine before entry into a boarding cattery, unless they have been vaccinated within the last 6 months.

Respiratory viruses are most prevalent in catteries, and household pets are most likely to be exposed when entering a boarding cattery or veterinary hospital. Therefore stress and contact with other cats should be avoided as far as possible, i.e. cat best cared for at home when owner on holiday.

Boarding catteries

All cats should have an up-to-date, fully completed vaccination record. In exceptional circumstances, where there is no alternative and rapid protection is required, the intranasal route may be used. However, the vaccine itself may cause mild clinical signs and the clients should be aware of this.

Cattery owners should not rely on vaccination alone, since virus will inevitably be present either from the occasional cat incubating the disease or from carriers.

Measures to prevent the spread of infection within a cattery are given in Table 1.3.

Stray cat homes

In general the same measures apply as with boarding catteries, but it is often impossible to separate animals to the same extent. Nevertheless, animals should be quarantined, or batched on arrival, and those with clinical signs isolated. Unless cats can be isolated on arrival for 3–4 weeks, the systemic vaccines may not have time to become effective. In these circumstances the intranasal route may be advisable: cats challenged 4 days after intranasal vaccination appear to be solidly immune, and some protection is present at 48 hours.

Breeding catteries

Disease-free colonies

- Vaccinate routinely if any contact, direct or indirect, with other cats.
- Inactivated vaccines are probably preferable. If attenuated live vaccines are used, care should taken in administering the vaccine.
- Avoid contact with carriers, i.e. avoid cats with any history of, or association with, oral or respiratory disease, remembering even vaccinated cats may be carriers, and kittens can become infected subclinically under cover of maternally derived antibody.
- Quarantine incoming cats for 3 weeks; ideally screen at least twice by means of an oropharyngeal swab for FCV (and FHV, though the intermittent shedding of this virus from carriers makes detection of this virus much less likely). If cats have never been vaccinated, serology can be done. Since FIV potentiates FCV infection, this should be tested for, and indeed FeLV, as well.

Table 1.3 Recommendations to prevent spread of the respiratory viruses in a boarding cattery

Make sure all incoming cats are fully vaccinated.

House cats individually, unless from same household.

Put cats with any signs of a previous respiratory infection (e.g. ocular discharge, chronic rhinitis), cats known to have had respiratory disease, and any suspect carrier cats from past experience in one section, or one end of the cattery and feed last – or do not accept for boarding.

Build cattery with solid partitions between pens. Ensure that frontages are at least 1 m apart, and that the surface of the pen is easily washable.

Arrange pen so food bowl and litter tray may be removed routinely without entering the pen, i.e. do not handle cats more than necessary.

Feed cats in same order every day and attend to each pen completely before moving on to the next.

Either: wash hands in disinfectant bucket between visiting each pen, or: have an individual pair of rubber gloves on a peg by each pen for use only with that pen. Disinfect thoroughly before use with a new boarder.

Wear rubber boots and step into a disinfectant bath if it is necessary to enter the pen.

Either: use disposable food trays or: have two sets of feed bowls used on alternate days. Soak used set in a 1 in 32 dilution of bleach in a solution of washing up liquid or in another appropriate disinfectant for several hours, and then leave thoroughly rinsed and dried until re-use 24 hours later.

Prepare food in central area.

Replace badly soiled litter trays with another previously disinfected and pre-filled in a central area, i.e. similar system to the feed bowls.

When cat goes home, thoroughly disinfect cage, allow to dry, and preferably leave empty for two days before re-using.

Reduce concentration of virus in environment by adequate ventilation, low relative humidity, optimum environmental temperatures.

Colonies with enzootic disease

In some circumstances it may be feasible to eliminate virus and with a barrier system maintain a virus-free colony. For example, an institutional colony could use specific-pathogen-free cats, and a pedigree cat breeding colony could use kittens from existing stock removed as soon as possible after birth and hand-reared in isolation. However, the viruses are very widespread, and it would be difficult to ensure that, even with vaccination, a colony would remain virus-free. For most situations, therefore, the only reasonable course is to attempt disease control. This may be done by the following:

- Carry out regular vaccination programmes.
- Give breeding queens boosters either prior to mating, or during pregnancy (with an inactivated vaccine only).
- Keep cats as stress-free as possible and employ good hygiene to reduce spread of viruses within colony.

- Avoid breeding from queens with a history of oral or respiratory disease in their kittens.
- Move queens into isolation to kitten at least 3 weeks before term so: kittens not exposed to shedding carriers in the colony, and if queen sheds virus as a result of the move, the episode will be over by the time the kittens are born.
- Wean kittens into isolation away from their mother as soon as feasible (ideally at 4–5 weeks well before maternal antibodies have waned), if it is likely she is a carrier.
- Vaccinate all kittens as soon as maternal antibodies are at a non-interfering level (normally 9+ weeks) and keep them in strict isolation until a week after the second dose.
- Earlier vaccination schedules may be used, the starting age being 7–10 days before the age in that particular colony when kittens first become affected.
  Both intranasal and systemic vaccines have been advocated:

  ○ Systemic vaccines may be given from 3 to 4 weeks of age, at 3 to 4-week intervals until 12 weeks.
  ○ Although not licensed for use in the UK in kittens less than 12 weeks of age, intranasal vaccine may be useful in young kittens as it may be better than some systemic vaccines at overcoming residual maternally derived antibody. Vaccination should be performed a week or so before disease has been occurring, and then again at 12 weeks: there is some evidence that multiple doses are not necessary although they were originally advocated. Vaccination of the queen via the intranasal route on the day of parturition has also been suggested.

FELINE *CHLAMYDIA PSITTACI* INFECTION

Feline *Chlamydia psittaci* infection occurs world-wide. The organism was originally thought to be the main cause of upper respiratory tract disease in the cat, which at that time was called 'feline pneumonitis'. Subsequently it became apparent that feline herpesvirus and feline calicivirus are the two main causes of feline respiratory disease: *C. psittaci* was found to be a conjunctival rather than a respiratory pathogen, and, despite the original name of feline pneumonitis, pneumonia does not generally occur.

AETIOLOGY

- Chlamydiae are highly specialised obligate intracytoplasmic bacteria. They have a rigid cell wall similar to Gram-negative bacteria, contain both DNA and RNA, and are susceptible to certain antibiotics.

- There are two main species within the genus *Chlamydia*: *C. trachomatis*, which generally only infects man, and *C. psittaci* which can infect many species of animals and birds causing respiratory disease, abortions and arthritis.
- Although many species of animals and birds are susceptible to *C. psittaci* infection, there are different strains of the organism with different tropisms, pathogenicity and host specificity, and genomic differences suggest that they should really be regarded as different species.
- Thus, the feline disease is caused by a feline strain of *C. psittaci*, and except for isolated reports of its possible involvement in human conjunctivitis, the organism is generally considered to be species specific. The only animal species from which isolates of *C. psittaci* appear to have a clearly established zoonotic potential are birds and sheep.

EPIDEMIOLOGY

- The disease tends to be more of a problem in colonies of cats.
- A UK survey has shown that 30% of swabs from cats with conjunctivitis were positive for *C. psittaci*. Infection was most common in kittens between 5 weeks and 9 months of age.
- Like the feline respiratory viruses, chlamydial infection is probably transmitted primarily by direct or fomite contact with infectious discharges, and possibly over short distances by aerosol.
- Chlamydiae, like the feline respiratory viruses, are relatively unstable outside their host, being inactivated by a number of lipid solvents and detergents.
- The organism is shed predominantly in conjunctival secretions: shedding from the conjunctivae has been demonstrated for up to 18 months after experimental infection. Chlamydiae have also been detected in vaginal and rectal swabs for several months after infection. The clinical and epidemiological significance of this is not known.
- Once the infection is enzootic in a colony, clinical signs may persist in some individuals for weeks, and recurrent episodes are common. It has been suggested that some of these recurrent episodes may be induced by stress, such as kittening and lactation, which may facilitate transmission of the organism between mothers and their kittens. However, there is some evidence that suckling kittens are usually protected from infection from their dam, presumably by colostrally derived antibodies, for the first 6 weeks of age.
- Thus, natural immunity to the disease appears to be relatively inefficient and incomplete, and infection appears to be perpetuated in a colony situation for some months, if not for years.

PATHOGENESIS AND CLINICAL SIGNS

- Conjunctival epithelium is the main target tissue for feline *C. psittaci*. However, the organism may also generalise, and has been found in gastric mucosa and in rectal and vaginal swabs.

- The incubation period ranges from 3 to 5 days experimentally to up to 14 days under natural conditions.
- The predominant clinical sign is a persistent conjunctivitis.
- Co-infection with the respiratory viruses, or secondary infection with bacteria or mycoplasmas, may lead to more severe disease, but generally, apart from marked conjunctival signs, the disease is mild.
- In the acute stages there is a marked serous ocular discharge (which later becomes mucopurulent) and blepharospasm, and the conjunctivae are hyperaemic and swollen.
- Initially only one eye may be affected, but usually both eyes eventually become involved.
- Mild nasal discharge, sneezing, and coughing may also occur, and there may be mild pyrexia in the initial stages of the disease. Affected cats generally stay well and continue to eat.
- Mild pulmonary lesions may be detected occasionally at necropsy, but pneumonitis is not usually apparent clinically.
- Follicular hyperplasia of the conjunctival lymphoid tissue has been reported, and corneal ulceration and keratitis have been described; however, it is probable that other agents, such as the respiratory viruses, were involved in such cases.
- Severe conjunctivitis generally persists for 3–4 weeks or so, but milder clinical signs may persist for some months: although most animals eventually recover, recurrent episodes may occur.
- Experimentally, there is some evidence that chlamydiae may infect the genital tract of cats, but the relevance of this to the field situation is not known. Although abortion has been noted in some cats infected with *C. psittaci*, in general it appears that *C. psittaci* is not involved in feline reproductive disease.

DIAGNOSIS

- Chlamydial infection may be diagnosed to a large extent on the characteristic clinical signs, specifically a marked, often persistent conjunctivitis (Table 1.1).
- Another aid in differentiation between chlamydial and viral infection of the respiratory tract is that chlamydial infection may respond to certain antibiotics (see below).
- Diagnosis may be confirmed in untreated cases by the following approaches:

  ○ A Giemsa-stained conjunctival scraping or smear may be directly examined for the presence of inclusion bodies. These are most numerous in the first 4–7 days of clinical disease, and are only occasionally seen up to 14 days. However, the results can be difficult to interpret.
  ○ More reliably, some specialist laboratories offer attempted isolation of the organism in cell culture from a firmly taken conjunctival swab. Chlamydiae are intracellular parasites, and it is important that epithelial

cells be present in the sample. Specialised transport media are required, and either rapid transport to the laboratory or −70°C storage before collection. Either immunofluorescence or histochemical stains can then be used to confirm the identify of the intracytoplasmic inclusions in the cell cultures.

○ Several commercial kits have been developed for use in diagnosis of human chlamydial infections and can be used for diagnosis in cats. These kits use a genus-specific monoclonal or polyclonal antibody which is either used in an immunofluorescent test on conjunctival smears, or has been incorporated into an ELISA. These techniques are not as sensitive as culture in the later stages of the disease, but have the advantage that both viable and non-viable organisms can be detected.

• In unvaccinated cats a positive serologic response or demonstration of a significant rise in antibody titre may also be helpful in diagnosis. The indirect immunofluorescent test is generally more reliable in detecting antibody than the older complement fixation test.

TREATMENT

• Although several antibiotics may have some effect on relieving the clinical signs of chlamydial infection, tetracyclines remain the drugs of choice.
• As systemic infection has been demonstrated it is probably advisable to treat both systemically and topically.
• Opthalmic ointment containing tetracycline should be applied 3–4 times daily. Currently only chlortetracycline is available in the UK.
• Oxytetracycline (20 mg/kg, 3 times daily) or doxycycline, a tetracycline derivative, (10 mg/kg, once a day), should be given systemically.
• All cats in the household should be treated simultaneously for at least 3–4 weeks or for at least 2 weeks after clinical signs have disappeared.
• Systemic tetracyclines are theoretically contraindicated in pregnant cats or in young kittens where there is calcification occurring. There is little evidence that treatment does, in fact, affect kittens' teeth but owners should be aware of the possibility.
• Erythromycin and tylosin may also be effective treatments, but no controlled trials have been carried out in cats.

PREVENTION AND CONTROL

• Because chlamydial infection is thought to be transmitted in a manner similar to that for the feline respiratory viruses, similar control measures to stop the spread of infection should apply.
• Because persistent or recurrent infection in a colony situation is common, it is important to treat all individuals in a cattery at the same time.

- Vaccination against feline *C. psittaci* infection has been employed in the USA for some years, and more recently in the UK and some other countries. Early vaccines were produced in eggs, but cell culture-derived vaccines have been developed. There has been some discussion as to the efficacy of the vaccines in the past. However, more recent studies have demonstrated significant (but not always complete) protection against disease but not necessarily against shedding. Protection appears to last for at least 1 year.
- Although there are only isolated case reports of possible zoonotic infection with the feline strain of *C. psittaci*, it is nevertheless wise to suggest taking hygiene precautions when handling or treating an infected pet.

BORDETELLA BRONCHISEPTICA INFECTION

HISTORY

- Originally associated with respiratory disease, particularly bronchopneumonia, in overcrowded conditions in mainly laboratory cats.
- More recently, associated with dyspnoea, cyanosis, pneumonia and death in a pedigree breeding colony.
- Signs of upper respiratory disease have now been seen in specific-pathogen-free cats (known to be free of the respiratory viruses) following both experimental inoculation and natural exposure.

Therefore it appears that *B. bronchiseptica* can act as both a primary and a secondary pathogen, though its precise role in the cases of respiratory disease in the field has yet to be determined.

PATHOGENESIS AND CLINICAL SIGNS

In dogs and other species *B. bronchiseptica* attaches to the cilia of the respiratory epithelium, thus overcoming the mucociliary clearance apparatus and allowing the bacteria to colonise the respiratory tract. In dogs this leads to tracheobronchitis, i.e. 'kennel cough'.

In studies in cats where *Bordetella* is known to be the sole pathogen, the following clinical signs may be seen:

- pyrexia
- sneezing
- nasal discharge
- mandibular lymphadenopathy

- spontaneous or induced coughing
- râles at auscultation.

In general, coughing is less of a feature of the disease in cats than in dogs.

Signs generally resolve after about 10 days.

Undoubtedly, combined infections with the respiratory viruses and stress factors such as weaning, overcrowding, poor hygiene and ventilation all play a role in *B. bronchiseptica* infections. Such factors may account for the severe cases of bronchopneumonia that have been reported in the field.

DIAGNOSIS

Differentiation on clinical signs alone is difficult (Table 1.1), and mixed infections are probably common. Bacterial isolation may be done from swabs taken from nasal discharge or from oropharyngeal secretions. Swabs should be transported in charcoal Amies transport medium and cultured on selective media such as charcoal–cephalexin agar (Oxoid, Unipath Ltd, UK).

TREATMENT

Oxytetracycline or doxycycline are the drugs of choice, although there is some evidence that oral administration of doxycycline may not eliminate shedding from carrier cats.

EPIDEMIOLOGY

- Infection is widespread in the cat population: a survey has shown that over 70% of 126 cats sampled were seropositive to *B. bronchiseptica* and the organism was isolated from approximately 5% of 527 cats tested. Infection appeared to be more common in multi-cat households with a history of respiratory disease.
- Some seropositive animals appear to be long-term carriers of the organism.
- Criteria for cat-to-cat transmission not yet established – some animals may shed higher levels of the bacterium and be of greater epidemiological significance.
- Inter-species transmission may be a possibility, e.g. between dogs and cats.

PREVENTION AND CONTROL

- Improve husbandry, i.e. good hygiene and ventilation, and minimise over-crowding.
- Vaccination may become available. A modified live intranasal vaccine is marketed for dogs, and an inactivated fimbrial subunit-based vaccine has been shown to work experimentally in cats.

MYCOPLASMA INFECTION

BACKGROUND

- The role of mycoplasmas in feline respiratory disease is not clear.
- Several species have been isolated from cats, the most common being *Mycoplasma felis* and *M. gatae*. Infection is common both in colony cats and household pets, and the organisms have been isolated from both diseased and healthy cats.
- *M. gatae* is probably a normal commensal of the conjunctivae and upper respiratory tract of cats and probably has little pathogenic potential for these sites.
- A pathogenic role has been suggested for *M. felis* in conjunctivitis and upper respiratory disease. Undoubtedly the organism can be important as a secondary pathogen, but evidence for its role as a primary pathogen is more equivocal. A higher isolation rate has been found for *M. felis* in some studies on cats with conjunctivitis and respiratory disease compared with normal cats, and some experimental studies have been done. Most of these studies are difficult to interpret however, as they have not been carried out in specific-pathogen-free cats and therefore other pathogens may have been involved.

CLINICAL SIGNS

The disease sign most often attributed to *M. felis* infection is a unilateral or bilateral conjunctivitis, with moderate to severe hyperaemia of both bulbar and palpebral conjunctivae and the nictitating membrane. Initially there is a serous discharge turning to mucopurulent discharge as the disease progresses. Signs generally resolve within 7–10 days.

DIAGNOSIS AND TREATMENT

Isolation of mycoplasmas requires specialised transport medium and culture conditions. A specialist laboratory is best contacted for guidance. In general, however, culture for mycoplasmas is not indicated. The organism is sensitive to several antibiotics including tetracycline and tylosin, but not to antibiotics such as penicillin which inhibit cell wall synthesis. Thus, in intractable cases of conjunctivitis where either *Chlamydia* or mycoplasmas might be involved, tetracycline is the drug of choice.

OTHER DISEASES CAUSED BY MYCOPLASMAS

M. gatae and *M. felis* have both been implicated in arthritis in cats, and bacterial L-forms have been associated both with joint disease and subcutaneous abscesses. Ureaplasmas have been implicated in one experimental study in spontaneous abortions and kitten mortality, but there is no evidence that this occurs in the field.

2 FELINE PANLEUCOPENIA

Feline panleucopenia (FP) is a highly infectious and ubiquitous disease affecting the domestic cat, other members of the Felidae (such as tiger, cheetah and leopard), the Mustellidae (e.g. mink and ferret), Procyonidae (e.g. coati-mundi, raccoon), and Viverridae (e.g. civet cat). The disease is characterised by a marked decrease in circulating white blood cells (i.e. a panleucopenia;) and destruction of the intestinal mucosa leading to enteritis. It was the first disease of the cat that was shown to be viral in origin. Vaccination is very effective, and in most situations the disease is now rare.

AETIOLOGY

- A parvovirus, a small (20 nm diameter) unenveloped, single-stranded DNA virus.
- Only one serotype known.
- Closely related to the recently emerged canine parvovirus, but minor differences do exist both in the viral DNA and antigenically.
- Parvoviruses have an affinity and requirement for actively dividing cells.
- Very stable virus in external environment; may survive in infected premises for up to a year.
- Susceptible to only a limited number of common disinfectants, e.g. hypochlorite, glutaraldehyde, or formaldehyde.

PATHOGENESIS

- May be predicted from the requirement of the virus for rapidly dividing cells (Figure 2.1).
- Main target organs are the crypt epithelium of the intestine, and lymphoid tissue and the bone marrow.

Intestinal effects

- Virus localises in crypt cells because these are most mitotically active.
- When crypt cells are destroyed by virus, no new cells are available to replace adsorptive cells at villus tips.

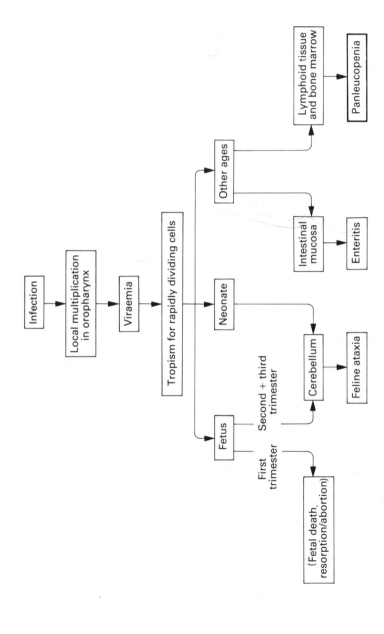

Figure 2.1 Pathogenesis of feline panleucopenia

- Therefore factors influencing mitotic rate of crypt cells (e.g. presence of bacterial flora, fasting) to some extent determine severity of disease.

Lymphoid tissue and bone marrow effects

- Virus attacks lymphocytes in lymphoid tissues, and leucocytic stem cells in bone marrow, leading to panleucopenia.
- Erythrocytopoiesis appears to remain unaltered; red cells survive longer anyway; therefore generally in the acute case, no anaemia present.

PATHOLOGY

Gross

- Changes often slight.
- Dehydration a feature.
- Evidence of vomiting or fetid diarrhoea.
- Jejunum and ileum dilated and oedematous with petechial haemorrhages ('rose-red' appearance) on the serosal and mucosal surfaces.
- Mesenteric lymph nodes may be oedematous and haemorrhagic.

Histopathology

Intestinal effects

- Lesions usually present in jejunum and ileum; sometimes also duodenum and colon.
- Mild to total destruction of epithelial lining, with dilatation of crypts.
- Crypts often filled with cellular debris.
- In early cases, transient intranuclear inclusion bodies may be seen.

Lymphoid tissue and bone marrow effects

- In *lymphoid tissues* lymphocytic depletion and reticulo-endothelial cell hyperplasia are regularly seen; mesenteric lymph nodes, Peyer's patches and spleen are particularly affected, and in younger animals also the thymus.
- In *bone marrow*, there is a general depression in myeloid activity with marked reduction in neutrophils and depletion of reticulum cell meshwork.

FELINE ATAXIA SYNDROME

- syndrome seen in young kittens
- virus infects and replicates in placental cells, and can then infect the fetus
- in first third of gestation infection → fetal death and resorption (Figure 2.1)
- from middle third of gestation to immediately post-natally infection → cerebellar hypoplasia (Figure 2.1)
- histologically, marked reduction in numbers of granular and Purkinje cells of cerebellum
- retina may also be affected, but not usually important clinically
- clinically, signs present at birth but not usually seen until walking age (2–3 weeks)
- not all the litter may be affected
- affected cats show symmetrical ataxia, a characteristic hypermetria, incoordination, and often intention tremors
- signs persist for life, but animal may compensate and thrive

CLINICAL SIGNS

The severity of the disease varies considerably in susceptible individuals, from either a subclinical infection, to a mild transient fever and leucopenia, to a severe, peracute syndrome where the cat may be found dead. In general, the disease tends to be more severe in young kittens.

The following signs are, however, often typical:

- Incubation period 2–10 days.
- First signs of illness are lethargy, fever, anorexia, and apparent thirst but refusal to drink.
- Vomiting generally occurs.
- Diarrhoea less common, particularly in early stages.
- Abdominal palpation reveals fluid-and-gas-filled intestines, and may elicit pain.
- After 2–3 days, symptoms variable, e.g. fever, profuse watery diarrhoea or dysentery, severe dehydration and electrolyte imbalance.
- Anaemia not usually present though may develop in long-standing cases especially if there is intestinal bleeding.
- Subnormal temperature carries grave prognosis.
- Mortality rate varies from 25% to 75%.
- Fatalities due to overwhelming bacterial infection, dehydration, and electrolyte imbalance.

DIAGNOSIS

- Presumptive diagnosis may be made on clinical signs, vaccination status, and also often on a history of recent possible exposure.
- Diagnosis may be confirmed by blood smear stained by Giemsa or methylene blue, and found to be nearly devoid of leucocytes.

- Laboratory haematology shows white blood counts below 7×10^9/litre, and often below 2×10^9/litre; after a week or so of illness a neutrophilia with a left shift may be present.
- In fatal cases gross post-mortem findings may be helpful. For histopathology, samples of jejunum and ileum, mesenteric lymph node and spleen should be taken into formal saline.
- Specialist virology laboratories can confirm the diagnosis, although false negatives do occur as the virus can be difficult to isolate.

  ○ From live animal: oropharyngeal swab, faeces, and, if possible, acute and convalescent sera should be sent by first class post.
  ○ From dead cat: fresh samples of spleen, mesenteric lymph node, ileum and faeces sent as above.

- Kits for the detection of canine parvovirus antigen in faeces may also detect FPV in faeces of many, but not all, cases of FP.

Differential diagnosis

- Presence of intestinal foreign bodies, especially if associated with obstruction or infection.
- Acute bacterial septicaemia.
- Toxoplasmosis.
- Poisoning.
- Occasionally, lymphosarcoma.
- Similar syndrome to FP, but associated with feline leukaemia virus infection, also described.

TREATMENT

Treatment should be supportive whilst the cat's own defences overcome the infection.

- Basically aimed at:

  ○ Controlling propensity for secondary bacterial infection.
  ○ Combating dehydration.
  ○ Restoring electrolyte imbalance.

- Treatment therefore consists of:

  ○ Parenteral, bactericidal, broad-spectrum antibiotic such as amoxycillin and clavulanic acid or a cephalosporin (since both gut absorption and the immune system are impaired).
  ○ Subcutaneous or intravenous fluids: 5% dextrose saline, lactated Ringer's solution or more complex balanced electrolyte solutions all suitable.
  ○ Whole blood: use equivocal as generally no anaemia. In early stages (< 5 days) may be useful as means of giving hyperimmune serum.

○ An anti-emetic, such as metoclopromide, may reduce fluid loss.
○ Oral and liquidised foods in later stages when gastro-intestinal signs have diminished. Low doses of diazepam can be used just before feeding to stimulate appetite.
○ Vitamin supplements.
○ Good nursing care: if treatment permits, home care best. (Remember marked resistance of virus to the environment and to many common disinfectants.)

EPIDEMIOLOGY

- Highly infectious
- In unvaccinated populations will be enzootic.
- Primarily a disease of young kittens as they lose maternal antibody.
- Morbidity generally 100%, but in many cases only mild or subclinical disease occurs.
- Seasonal incidence with summer and autumn peaks noted in some areas because of seasonal birth rate.

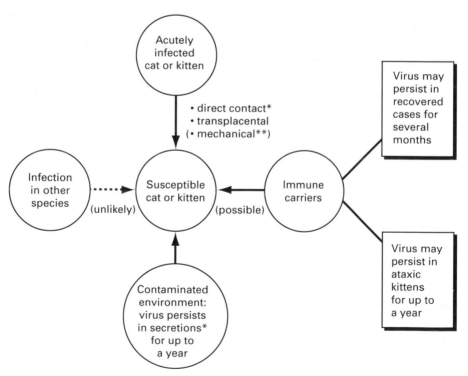

* Virus present in large quantities in saliva, urine, faeces and vomitus.
** For example, biting and flying insects, but unlikely to be of any significance.

Figure 2.2 Epidemiology of FP

The virus is perpetuated in the cat population in three main ways (Figure 2.2):

(1) By contact spread from acutely infected to susceptible animals; this depends on sufficient numbers of susceptible animals in the population and sufficient opportunities for contact between them.
(2) By persisting in the recovered cat, i.e. immune carriers.
(3) By persisting in the environment.

Of these, (1) and (3) are by far the most important.

VACCINATION AND CONTROL

- one serotype
- highly antigenic } both natural and vaccine induced immunity high and long-lived.

Vaccination has been very successful where it has been carried out.

Both modified live and inactivated systemic vaccines are available. Both confer perfectly adequate immunity, though modified live vaccines may induce slightly greater and possibly more rapid protection. Inactivated vaccines can, however, be used safely in pregnant queens and, if necessary, in young kittens, and are free from the, albeit small, risk of contamination from extraneous agents or reversion to virulence.

In kittens born to immune queens there is a high degree of correlation between antibody titres in queens and passive immunity levels in kittens. However, although a normagraph has been devised to predict at what age successful vaccination may be performed, in general for FP such an individual approach is not necessary. This is probably because in most breeding colonies immunity is usually in a reasonably steady state as a result of a long tradition of effective vaccination and absence of clinical disease.

For vaccination purposes, kittens may therefore be divided empirically into the categories shown in Table 2.1.

Duration of immunity

Thought to be relatively long. Thus:

- Cats that have had natural disease have very high serum neutralising antibody titres.
- Cats vaccinated with attenuated vaccines have moderate titres, which have been shown to persist for at least 4 years.
- Cats vaccinated with inactivated vaccines have slightly lower titres, but these also persist for at least a year.

On balance, initial booster advocated at one year, plus further doses at 1 to 2-yearly intervals, depending on the type of vaccine used and likelihood of exposure, e.g. entry into a boarding cattery. Natural exposure and boosting may occur, but cannot be relied upon.

Table 2.1 Vaccination regimes

1	Kittens born to mothers with moderate titres acquired through vaccination.	Lose their maternally derived immunity at 8–12 weeks.	(a) Vaccinate at 12 weeks if little risk of exposure and can keep isolated until vacc. immunity develops. (b) Vaccinate at 8–9 weeks if exposure likely, with second dose 3–4 weeks later.
2	Kittens born to mothers with high titres as a result of exposure to virulent virus, or vaccinated with live virus just before or during pregnancy.	Maternally derived immunity may persist for 16 weeks.	As above but extra dose at 16 weeks plus.
3	Kittens presented at 12 weeks of age with unknown vaccination status.		Generally one dose sufficient but additional dose at 16 weeks if category (2) suspected.
4	Kittens born to mothers where inadequate maternally derived antibody suspected and exposure likely.		Vaccinate at 4–6 (inactivated vaccine), 8 and 12 weeks of age.

Vaccination breakdowns and control

A regular vaccination programme, as outlined above, should ensure a good level of protection in most animals. In addition, cats on first entering a colony should be vaccinated fully at least 2 weeks before entry, and quarantined for 2–3 weeks on arrival. In boarding catteries, all cats should be housed individually, with their own equipment and utensils, and any animals with suspect clinical signs kept strictly isolated and fed last.

Nevertheless in open colonies and even in well controlled colony situations, breakdowns may sometimes still occur. This may be because of, for example:

- Lapses in vaccination schedules.
- Intercurrent disease (e.g. with FeLV, FIV).
- Individual immunological incompetence.
- Overwhelming infection from a clinical case.
- Kittens who are unprotected because they have just lost their maternally derived antibody (MDA), or they were vaccinated whilst MDA was still present at an interfering level.

Once even one case has occurred, the environment will be heavily contaminated, and this may then lead to further cases.

Thus:

- All pens, bedding, feeding and cleaning utensils, clothing and footwear of personnel should be adequately cleansed and disinfected.
- Booster vaccinations should be given to all cats, and inactivated vaccine to any pregnant queen.
- Following adequate disinfection, a cat fully vaccinated 2 weeks previously may be safely introduced on to the premises.
- Where disinfection is difficult (e.g. in a house), or a replacement kitten is too young for the vaccination course to be completed, it might be advisable to wait for several months, or to confine the cat to different quarters.

3   FELINE CORONAVIRUS INFECTION

THE VIRUSES

Feline coronaviruses; (FCoV) are often divided into two groups:

- the highly pathogenic strains, feline infectious peritonitis viruses (FIPV); and
- those strains which cause mild or no disease, the feline enteric coronaviruses (FECV).

FIPV and FECV are very closely related, and it has been suggested that FECV and FIPV strains comprise the extremes of a single population of viruses with a spectrum of pathogenicity. However, evidence is accumulating that FIPV strains may be mutants of FECV which arise spontaneously during infection.

Canine coronavirus (CCV), which causes diarrhoea in dogs, is also infectious to cats, and cats may develop antibody reactive with CCV and FCoV after contact with dog faeces containing CCV. CCV is very closely related antigenically and at the genome level to the feline coronaviruses.

PATHOGENESIS

The outcome of coronavirus infection in domestic cats depends on the strain and dose of virus, and the age, immune competence and immune status of the cat. In particular, the ability of the cat to mount a strong cell-mediated immune (CMI) response to the virus is believed to be very important in determining the clinical sequelae to infection. Thus infection can cause a wide spectrum of disease, or, very often, no disease at all (Figure 3.1).

- Main route of virus entry is oronasal, leading to virus replication in the oropharynx and in the enterocytes at the tips of villi. Experimentally, cats can also be infected via the respiratory tract with aerosols. There is also some evidence of transplacental transmission although this is not common in the field and appears to play little role in the overall epidemiology of feline coronavirus infection.
- If the cat mounts a strong immune response, particularly a strong cell-mediated immune response and a good local immune response in the gut, or

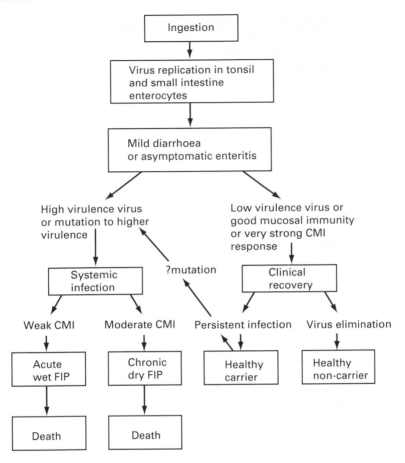

Figure 3.1 Probable pathogenesis of FIP

the virus is of low pathogenicity, then virus replication will be limited to the gut, and clinical signs will be absent or limited to mild diarrhoea.
- If the cell-mediated immune response is not so strong, then a more pathogenic virus may escape from the gut, giving rise to systemic infection. More pathogenic viruses are especially able to grow in macrophages, and it is in macrophages and monocytes that virus is disseminated.
- If a moderate cell-mediated immune response is encountered, then the development of lesions is slow, giving rise to chronic, dry feline infectious peritonitis.
- If, however, the cat produces a still weaker cell-mediated immune response, then acute, wet FIP rapidly develops.

This *model for the pathogenesis* of feline coronavirus infection explains why cats with wet FIP often have some lesions of dry FIP at necropsy, and also explains anecdotal accounts of cats recovering from wet FIP, but going on to develop dry FIP, or even (rarely) to recover.

It also explains why concurrent FeLV infection increases the prevalence of clinical FIP in a colony with FCoV infection, and suggests that treatments involving immunosuppressive agents, e.g. corticosteroids, although they might provoke a short-term general improvement in the cat's demeanour, would depress the CMI response and cause more severe disease in the long run.

The role of antibody

The role of antibody in the pathogenesis of FIP is complex. Local antibody in the gut appears to be protective but, experimentally at least, circulating, humoral IgG may cause enhancement of disease. The mechanism of antibody enhancement is not known, although it may involve antibody-mediated opsonisation without inactivation of the virus. This would increase the amount of virus which gets into macrophages, which are one of the major target cells for virus infection.

Carriers

Rather than overt clinical disease or virus elimination, some cats become persistently infected virus carriers. The mechanisms of persistent coronavirus infection and rates of excretion are not known, but these cats, particularly carrier queens, obviously play an important role in the epidemiology of FCoV infection.

CLINICAL SIGNS

Infection with FCoV is associated with several clinical syndromes in the field, although in most cases no clinical signs are observed.

Enteritis associated with low-virulence coronavirus (e.g. FECV) infection is generally mild and transient. It is most common in kittens, particularly just after weaning. More severe diarrhoea has been reported, but is rare. Some cats infected with more pathogenic strains of FCoV also have mild, transient diarrhoea several weeks before developing FIP.

The initial signs of both dry and wet FIP are rather non-specific and often missed in field cases. Cats may be pyrexic, inappetant, depressed and lethargic. Occasionally, mild diarrhoea may develop.

Dry FIP

In dry FIP, granulomatous lesions develop in a variety of organs and the clinical signs reflect the organs involved.

- Most frequently affected are organs in the abdominal cavity, particularly the liver and kidney.

- Other common sites include the central nervous system (dry FIP is the most common lesion of the CNS in necropsy surveys) and eye.
- The most common presenting signs are therefore chronic pyrexia, weight loss and depression if abdominal organs are most affected.
- Lesions in the central nervous system may lead to a variety of neurological signs including ataxia, paresis or paralysis, nystagmus, fits and behavioural changes, and lesions in the eye often present as uveitis.

Wet FIP

Wet FIP is characterised by the development of ascites with weight loss, depression, anaemia and death.

- As well as ascites, pleural and pericardial effusion occurs in about 20% of cases and in these cats dyspnoea is a prominent clinical sign.
- Jaundice is also sometimes seen, especially in the later stages of disease.
- Some cats may also have uveitis, and small granulomatous lesions more typical of dry FIP may be found at necropsy.

Although FIP is often thought of as two discrete syndromes, wet and dry FIP are not mutually exclusive descriptions. Eye or CNS lesions may be clinically apparent in up to 10% of cases of wet FIP and many cats with wet FIP have some lesions of dry FIP at necropsy. There are also occasional accounts of cats with wet FIP apparently recovering but then developing dry FIP.

FIP IN CHEETAHS

There have been several reports of outbreaks of FIP in captive cheetahs. The mortality rates in these outbreaks was fairly high, and it has been suggested that cheetahs might be particularly susceptible genetically to coronavirus infection. However, similarly high mortality rates have been reported in some domestic cat outbreaks and convincing evidence of special susceptibility in cheetahs is lacking.

DIAGNOSIS

Diagnosis of past coronavirus infection is simple, but diagnosis of FIP, the carrier state or active enteric infection may be very difficult.

Clinical signs

- Mild, transient enteritis, especially in kittens, can have many causes, but a rising antibody titre to FCoV might incriminate coronaviruses, and electron microscopy of faeces might help detect FECV or other viral causes.

- Acute, wet FIP in which the main sign is ascites is fairly obvious, although lymphocytic cholangitis can produce identical clinical signs, with proteinaceous ascitic fluid.
- Because dry FIP may present as a variety of syndromes, including renal failure, hepatitis or neurological signs, dry FIP is more difficult to diagnose in the live cat.

Differential diagnosis

Wet FIP

peritonitis	abdominal/thoracic neoplasia
heart failure	hepatic cirrhosis
pyothorax	chylothorax
lymphocytic cholangitis	cystic kidney
pregnancy	pyometra

Dry FIP

feline leukaemia virus	feline immunodeficiency virus
toxoplasmosis	neoplasia
cryptococcosis	

renal failure, hepatic disease, signs of CNS disease

Always suspect dry FIP in chronically ill, wasting cats, or cats with signs of CNS disease.

Clinical pathology

Serum

	FIP	Normal
Increased total serum protein	>80 g/l	60–80 g/l
Increased serum globulin	>50 g/l	25–50 g/l
Decreased serum albumin:globulin ratio	<0.5	0.5–1.0

Increased bilirubin or urea and enzymes associated with renal or hepatic disease.

Depends on which organs most affected, e.g. in dry FIP may see elevated serum alkaline phosphatase (SAP) and serum glutamic transaminase (SGPT) associated with hepatic lesions. In acute wet FIP may see jaundice (but often without elevated SAP and SGPT).

Peritoneal fluid

In cats with wet FIP, the peritoneal fluid:

- is clear/slightly cloudy, straw-yellow in colour;
- has high protein concentration (foams when shaken) (50–100 g/l);
- clots on exposure to air;
- has few leucocytes (cf. septic peritonitis).

Haematology

Variable and fairly non-specific changes. May include:

	FIP	*Normal range*
Decreased PCV	<30%	(30–45%)
Decreased RBC	$<5 \times 10^{12}/l$	$(5–10 \times 10^{12}/l)$
Increased WBC	$>5 \times 10^{12}/l$	$(5–15 \times 10^{9}/l)$
Increased neutrophils	65–90%	(35–75%)
Decreased lymphocytes	<8%	(12–30%)

Virus isolation

Virus isolation is not usually possible from field cases. This is partly because virus is not shed uniformly throughout the course of the disease (making it difficult to know which samples to take and when to take them) but mainly because most field strains are difficult, if not impossible, to grow in cell culture. Several techniques for detecting virus without having to grow it are being investigated, in particular ELISAs for circulating antigen or immune complexes and polymerase chain reaction assays for use on various tissues and faeces, but none is as yet commercially available.

Serological assays

Serological assays are the laboratory tests most used to help diagnose FCoV infection, but are difficult to interpret. ELISA kits are available for use in the practice laboratory, although, at the time of writing, we find that immuno-fluorescence (IF) tests, as done by most feline virus diagnostic laboratories, are more sensitive. The results of serological tests for FCoV infection should be interpreted with care.

Interpretation of FIP serology

It is important to remember that serological tests can only detect detectable antibody – and the amount of detectable antibody to FCoV circulating in a cat does not correlate very well with disease.

Thus absence of antibody does not preclude acute wet FIP – possibly because acutely ill cats have so much circulating antigen that it binds all the antibody leaving none free for detection.

Detectable antibody at any titre merely indicates either past or present infection. Cats with dry FIP generally have high antibody titres ($\geqslant$ 320), but high antibody titres may also be found in healthy, recovered cats.

As antibody titres generally decline following virus elimination, cats with persistent antibody should be treated as suspect virus carriers; however, it may be that some cats with no detectable antibody can also be virus carriers.

Histopathology

At present, the only way of making a definitive diagnosis of FIP is by histopathological examination of diseased tissues. Such tissues may be taken at necropsy or biopsy, e.g. of liver in wet FIP or of other affected organs in dry FIP.

- The histological lesions of wet and dry FIP include fibrinous deposits and small pyogranulomas on the omentum and serosal surfaces of most abdominal organs.
- Perivascular cuffing is often seen both within the serosa and along venules in underlying tissues.
- Follicular hyperplasia, necrotic foci and pyogranulomatous lesions are commonly found in abdominal lymph nodes and the spleen.
- Dry FIP involves similar histopathological changes to those of wet FIP although the granulomatous lesions are usually much larger and are surrounded by more fibrosis, and are often found outside the abdomen and thorax – particularly in the CNS and eye.

EPIDEMIOLOGY (Figure 3.2)

FIP is most frequently seen in young kittens raised in colonies, although occasional cases are also seen in older pet cats. The main sources of infection within a colony in which FCoV infection is enzootic appear to be carrier queens. The virus is passed on to their kittens before weaning, and these infected kittens may be a further source of infection to other kittens in the colony. In coronavirus-free colonies, or among pet cats which do not meet other cats very often, the main source of infection is other carrier, or acutely infected, cats.

Cats may also be infected with canine coronavirus through contact with dog faeces, although the role of CCV in FIP in the field is not known.

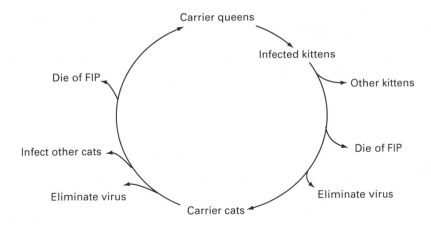

Figure 3.2 FIP epidemiology

TREATMENT

- No effective specific treatment exists for FIP.
- Antivirals (e.g. ribavirin) and immunomodulators (e.g. interferons) inhibit virus production in cell culture but have little or no effect in cats.
- Use of antibiotics and corticosteroids may relieve some clinical signs temporarily, but not in the long term.
- Some cats recover spontaneously (very rare).
- Good nursing, symptomatic treatment and draining of ascitic fluid from cats with wet FIP may alleviate the clinical signs in some cats, sometimes for several months, although these cats may develop dry FIP later.

CONTROL

Vaccination

There have been many attempts to develop an effective vaccine against FIP. Experimentally, killed and attenuated vaccines have generally failed through the phenomenon of *antibody enhancement* of disease (see 'Pathogenesis').

Use of related viruses such as CCV as vaccines has caused either no protection or enhancement of subsequent infection, and genetically engineered vaccines expressing only one of each of the three main structural proteins of FCoV have similarly caused either enhancement or no protection.

However, a temperature-sensitive mutant has been licensed for use in North America and some EU countries (Primucell, Pfizer). This vaccine strain replicates only in the oropharynx where the temperature is lower than the rest of the body and, by producing a good mucosal immunity but only minimal systemic antibody, is thought to provoke protection without enhancement. Most experimental and field data suggest that the vaccine is both safe and probably effective. Experimental data suggest that under some conditions it might provoke enhancement of subsequent infection, but this has not been seen following natural challenge.

Control of infection

In a coronavirus-free colony, test all cats before they enter the colony, and do not take seropositive cats. If possible, ensure that cats entering the colony come from colonies where all the cats are seronegative. Quarantine all cats entering the colony for 12 weeks, and test again for antibody. Do not forget dogs as a possible source of infection.

In a colony with FCoV infection, isolate queens with their kittens for 12 weeks, and then test kittens. Do not allow seropositive kittens back into the colony. Early weaning and removal of kittens from seropositive queens can enable eradication of infection from a colony. Similarly, although there is evidence to suggest that occasional carrier cats may be seronegative, in practice removal of seropositive cats from the colony will often eradicate infection.

4 FELINE LEUKAEMIA VIRUS INFECTION

AETIOLOGY

- Caused by a retrovirus in the type-C oncornavirus subfamily.
- Three subtypes of virus – A, B and C – can be distinguished serologically and by genome analysis. Only FeLV-A is transmissible between cats.

FeLV-B, which is only found in cats also infected with FeLV-A, arises through recombination between type A virus and endogenous FeLV. FeLV-C is the least common subtype encountered and is also only found in cats infected with FeLV-A. FeLV-C strains appear to be mutants of FeLV-A.

PATHOGENESIS (Figure 4.1)

- The main route of virus infection is by ingestion although transplacental transmission also occurs.
- Virus is excreted in saliva, urine, faeces and milk, and close contact and licking are the usual means of spread.

FeLV replicates in the oropharynx, particularly the tonsils, from which it is spread to other lymphoid tissues, especially bone marrow. Many cats mount an immune response which eliminates the virus at this stage although latent infection of the bone marrow can still occur.

More extensive virus replication in the bone marrow can give rise to viraemia and widespread infection, especially in lymphoid tissues and epithelial cells of the oropharynx, salivary glands and upper respiratory tract, with consequent virus excretion and transmission to other cats. At this stage an effective immune response can still eliminate active infection, giving rise to a transient viraemia lasting between 2 days and 8 weeks.

Some cats, however, will not eliminate virus but develop persistent infection. It is persistently infected cats that will go on to develop clinical disease and which are the main source of infection to other cats.

The extent and clinical outcome of infection vary according to the age of the cat, its pre-existing immunity and the dose of virus received.

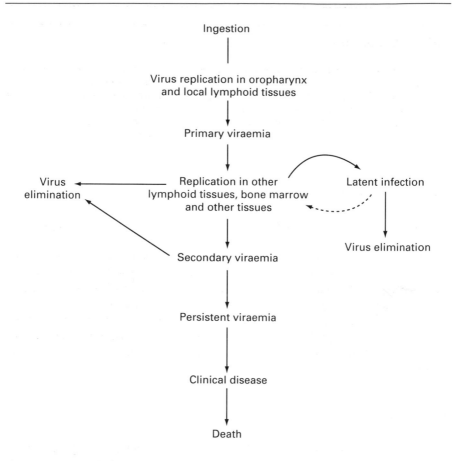

Figure 4.1 Pathogenesis of FeLV infection

- The susceptibility of kittens to infection decreases markedly with age such that persistent infection develops in only about one in five cats over 16 weeks old.
- Virus neutralising antibody in colostrum may protect kittens for the first 4 weeks of life.
- The dose of virus received depends largely on the kittens' environment:

  ○ In free-range cats the amount of contact between excreting and susceptible cats is small; the dose is therefore small. Although most cats will be infected, very few develop persistent infection.
  ○ In multi-cat households, however, the degree of contact and therefore exposure to virus is high, and in this situation up to 30% of kittens can become persistently infected.
  ○ A persistently infected queen will usually result in persistent infection in all the kittens in her litter.

Latent infection

Up to half of those cats which apparently recover from FeLV infection undergo latent infection in bone marrow. Virus release from latent infections is generally too low to be detected or to infect epithelial cells, and latently infected cats are therefore rarely sources of infection to other cats. Latent virus can, however, be induced to replicate by, for example, corticosteroid treatment. Even latent infections are usually eliminated, although around 10% of cats can remain latently infected for at least three years.

CLINICAL SIGNS

FeLV infection is probably the most common infectious cause of death in young adult cats.

Clinical disease is seen in persistently infected cats, most of which will die within 4 years of meeting the virus. The clinical syndromes associated with FeLV infection are mainly associated with infection of the haemopoietic system. Infection of the bone marrow can have severe effects on the development of both lymphoid and myeloid cells giving rise to proliferation (neoplasia) or depression, although the precise mechanisms of pathogenesis are often not known. In addition, FeLV infection is often associated with reproductive failure.

Neoplasia

FeLV can cause neoplasia of lymphoid or myeloid tissue, although the most common haemopoietic malignancy in the cat is lymphosarcoma, which accounts for 90% of haemopoietic tumours and around one-third of all feline neoplasia. Most cases of lymphosarcoma in the cat are associated with FeLV infection.

Lymphosarcoma can be divided into four main types.

Thymic (anterior mediastinal) lymphosarcoma

- Mainly in younger cats (<3 years old).
- T-cells in thymus +/− local lymph nodes; seldom in blood.
- Signs include tachypnoea, dyspnoea, regurgitation and weight loss.
- Often pleural fluid (→ muffled heart sounds) containing neoplastic cells (cytology of aspirates).
- Often can palpate increased thoracic resistance.
- Diagnosis by radiography, cytology of pleural effusion, biopsy of mass, 80% FeLV positive.

Multicentric lymphosarcoma

- Peripheral gross lymphadenopathy and enlarged spleen.
- Often mild anaemia.
- Average age 4 years.
- Diagnosis by biopsy, 60% FeLV positive.

Alimentary lymphosarcoma

- Abdominal masses (mainly between duodenum and colon – rarely stomach or rectum), sometimes more diffuse.
- Often involves local lymph nodes, occasionally kidney.
- Anorexia, weight loss, vomiting if high obstruction, sometimes diarrhoea, often anaemic.
- Average age 8 years.
- Diagnosis by clinical signs, abdominal palpation, radiography, laparotomy. Only 30% FeLV positive.

Lymphoid leukaemia

- Based in bone marrow and affects also haematopoiesis.
- Therefore raised WBC, anaemia and, often, thrombocytopenia (with petechial haemorrhages on skin and mucous membranes).
- Pyrexia, weakness, loss of appetite.
- Often enlarged spleen but rarely enlarged lymph nodes.
- Diagnosis by haematology (neoplastic cells in smear), marrow biopsy/aspirate, FeLV positive in 60% cases.

Lymphosarcomas are also frequently found in the kidney, nose, eye, CNS and skin.

FeLV-negative lymphosarcoma

FeLV-negative lymphosarcoma may be nothing to do with FeLV; for example, may be primary neoplastic events or possibly due to FIV infection in older cats. However, FeLV-negative cases of lymphosarcoma are more common in cats from colonies with enzootic FeLV infection, so it may be that in these cases the cat's immune response eliminated the virus, but only after transformation of some cells had already occurred.

Myeloid leukaemia

Myeloid leukaemia is uncommon. May involve granulocytes or erythroid cells. Primary lesion is in bone marrow, with possible secondaries in liver, spleen and lymph nodes. Generally progressive anaemia, intermittent pyrexia and weight loss. Thrombocytopenia causes petechial haemorrhage, and leucopenia causes immunosuppression and secondary infections. Diagnosis is by biopsy and haematology. Almost always FeLV positive, but eosinophilic leukaemia is usually FeLV negative.

Anaemia

Anaemia is relatively common in cats compared with other species, and FeLV infection is probably the most important cause. The anaemia may be primary or the result of lymphoid or myeloid leukaemia interfering with normal haematopoiesis. Primary red cell aplasia causes rapid onset anaemia. The packed cell volume may drop below 10%, although white cell counts remain normal. Because the anaemia is non-regenerative, RBCs are normocytic and normochromic.

A mild, often missed, haemolytic anaemia may also be common in FeLV-infected cats.

Total marrow aplasia is rare. Affected cats have severe leucopenia and anaemia, giving rise to rapid onset weight loss, anorexia and pyrexia. At necropsy these cats may have a haemorrhagic enteritis and haemorrhagic mesenteric lymph nodes.

Immunosuppression

The pathogenic mechanism underlying FeLV-induced immunosuppression is complex and not well understood. The strain of virus is important, and there may be a role for the envelope protein, p15E, which can inhibit lymphocyte growth *in vitro*. Immunosuppressed cats are susceptible to various secondary infections, and the clinical signs associated with FeLV immunosuppression are therefore varied.

- Cats persistently infected with FeLV are particularly susceptible to viral, bacterial and fungal respiratory and enteric infections and enteritis. Such cats are often thin and chronically ill, or have persistent pyrexia.
- May be associated with gingivitis and stomatitis, although in older cats this syndrome is more likely to be associated with feline immunodeficiency virus infection.
- *Haemobartonella* infection and anaemia is more common in FeLV-infected cats than non-infected cats.
- Clinical feline infectious peritonitis is more common in colonies with FeLV.
- Persistent abscessation or prolonged healing times in young cats may also be due to FeLV immunosuppression.
- An FeLV-associated 'panleucopenia-like' enteritis has also been reported, although it has been suggested that this may be linked to undetected feline parvovirus infection.

Reproductive failure

- FeLV infection is a common cause of reproductive failure in cats.
- Resorption of fetus usually occurs at 3–5 weeks into pregnancy, so pregnancy may have been confirmed by palpation of small fetal swellings.

- Resorption may be accompanied by a slight vulval discharge.
- Affected queens will often have had normal pregnancies previously.
- The mechanism of fetal death is not known, but may be due to placentitis or endometritis.
- If the fetuses survive to term, then the kittens will be persistently infected and are often sickly: FeLV is therefore a possible cause of fading kitten syndrome.

TREATMENT

Treatment of FeLV-related anaemias, immunosuppression and reproductive failure involves non-specific, supportive therapy only and carries a very poor prognosis.

Little success has been reported for treatments of either lymphatic or myeloid leukaemias. Remission rates of up to 60% for 2 years can be achieved by treatment of thymic and multicentric lymphosarcomas, although these cats will still be infected with FeLV and are therefore likely to develop another FeLV-related disease and be a source of infection to other cats.

Various treatment regimes using combinations of cytotoxic drugs and corticosteroids have been reported. However, as correct dosage and monitoring of patients are critical and as many of the protocols are complex, it is advisable either to refer the cat to a specialist centre or to take specialist advice before embarking on chemotherapy.

DIAGNOSIS

Several companies make and market ELISA or similar assays to test whole blood, serum, plasma or saliva for FeLV antigen. Infection should be confirmed by virus isolation or by immunofluorescence as some cats may be positive by ELISA but negative by virus isolation as antigen can occasionally be present in the circulation although virus infection has been eliminated from the blood. In addition, ELISA kits may sometimes give false positive results, for example, if the cat serum sample has haemolysed. Cats should be retested after 12 weeks to determine whether the viraemia is transient or persistent.

CONTROL

Test-and-remove

Routine testing followed by removal of any FeLV-infected cats has enabled many colonies to eradicate infection. The protocol used is fairly simple and not too expensive.

- Test all cats, and separate FeLV positive from negative; no additions to either group, and disinfect housing, etc.

- Retest after 12 weeks – remove all positives (kill or rehouse).
- Retest all cats every 6–12 months.
- Test, isolate for 12 weeks and retest all introductions to colony.

Vaccination

Several sub-unit and killed vaccines are available. Published reports show that the vaccines appear safe and provide good protection in most experimental challenges.

- Vaccination is recommended for use in cats from 9 weeks of age.
- Some veterinary surgeons recommend routine testing for FeLV antigenaemia prior to vaccination as the vaccine will not eliminate pre-existing infection. However, the cost of such testing needs to be weighed against risk of vaccine apparent failure.
- Vaccination does *not* cause an antigenaemia and therefore does *not* interfere with standard FeLV antigen assays. Thus the detection of FeLV viraemia or antigenaemia in a vaccinated cat must be due to natural infection, not the vaccine.
- Because the vaccines are not live, the immunity they provide is not life-long (unlike that often afforded by natural infection) and annual booster vaccination is recommended. Since most cats over 5 years old will have met natural FeLV infection and developed a good immune response to the virus, the benefits versus cost of vaccination of older cats might be considered on an individual basis.
- Although a large market exists for FeLV vaccination among pet cats housed singly, probably it is most useful in breeding colonies where FeLV infection is, or might potentially be, a problem.
- In such a situation, routine vaccination of all cats, but especially young kittens, will help prevent and control any outbreak without interfering with routine testing or posing any risk of vaccine-induced infection.
- However, because, like most other vaccines, FeLV vaccines cannot provide 100% protection, they should only be used as an adjunct to, not a replacement for, test-and-remove schemes.
- It is important to remember that vaccination does not guarantee that the cat is free from FeLV. It may therefore be a possible source of infection to other cats.

FELINE SARCOMA VIRUS

Feline sarcoma viruses (FeSV) arise through recombination of FeLV with parts of the host cell genome. This results in the formation of recombinant viruses which have deletions rendering them unable to replicate without the help of wild-type FeLV, but which contain a cellular oncogene and are capable of causing tumours, mainly of fibroblastic cells.

FeSV has been reported world-wide but is rare. FeSV tumours are seen only in cats persistently infected with FeLV. As the tumours contain FeLV and FeSV, the tumours are transmissible experimentally, but there is no evidence that natural cat-to-cat transmission occurs. FeSV is found almost entirely in the tumour itself, and only wild-type FeLV is shed from affected cats.

Tumours appear usually as multiple, ulcerative or nodular, non-healing skin lesions, which recur after surgical excision. Metastasis to internal organs may occur late in the course of the disease. All affected cats are FeLV antigenaemic. Unlike spontaneous fibrosarcomas of cats, which are usually solitary and seen in older cats, most FeSV-induced tumours are seen in cats 1–7 years old.

Diagnosis is usually based on history, FeLV status and histological confirmation of fibrosarcoma, although complete confirmation of the diagnosis requires extensive laboratory studies.

5 FELINE IMMUNODEFICIENCY VIRUS INFECTION

AETIOLOGY

Feline immunodeficiency virus (FIV) is a lentivirus (retrovirus family). It is related structurally, biochemically and by nucleotide sequence to human immuno-deficiency virus (HIV), the cause of AIDS in man, and infection of cats is also often associated with eventual development of clinically apparent immuno-deficiency. FIV does not infect human cells, and repeated surveys have shown no evidence of human infection with FIV.

EPIDEMIOLOGY

- FIV has been detected in domestic cats world-wide.
- FIV can be isolated from most antibody-positive domestic cats.
- Antibody to FIV-like viruses has also been detected in other species of cat both in the wild and in zoological collections, although there are few isolates from non-domestic cats.
- The prevalence of antibody in domestic cats varies with the lifestyle and age of the cats; generally about 20% of random 'sick cats' have antibody to FIV compared with less than 5% of healthy cats.
- Infection is more common in male domestic cats than in females, and most infected cats are over 5 years old.
- FIV infection is more common in free-roaming cats, feral cats, and cats which live in unstable colonies. Antibody can be detected in about one-third of cats in contact with an infected cat.

The main route of transmission is believed to be by inoculation of virus when biting. Large amounts of virus can be isolated from saliva, and transmission by biting has been demonstrated experimentally. Transplacental spread to fetuses has been demonstrated experimentally, but the occasional cases of spread from queens to kittens probably result from horizontal (e.g. virus in saliva or milk) transmission.

- The biting theory of transmission fits in with the epidemiology of FIV infec-tion: high-risk groups are adult, male, free roaming or live in unstable colonies.

- Pedigree breeding colonies are generally more stable, with less fighting and a lower prevalence of infection.

CLINICAL SIGNS

Following experimental inoculation of kittens with FIV, lymphadenopathy, sometimes accompanied by mild pyrexia, depression and leucopenia, usually develops after about 4 weeks. This lymphadenopathy can be less severe in older cats, however, and is therefore usually missed in naturally infected cats. The lymphadenopathy gradually disappears after a few weeks to months.

Infected cats can then remain healthy for years before clinical FIV-related disease is seen. Indeed many cats probably die of other causes long before AIDS-like disease develops.

- Clinical disease associated with FIV infection is seen mainly in middle-aged or elderly cats.
- Like AIDS in man, clinical signs are often caused not directly by FIV but by secondary infections often with micro-organisms which in an immuno-competent animal would cause only mild, if any, disease.

The clinical syndromes most often associated with FIV infection are:

- chronic stomatitis and severe gingivitis
- chronic upper respiratory tract disease
- wasting
- pyrexia
- lymphadenopathy
- anaemia
- chronic skin disease
- chronic diarrhoea
- neurological signs.

- Neurological disease is thought to be caused directly by FIV infection of the CNS. FIV-related neurological disease may present as motor or sensory deficits or as behavioural changes, including abnormalities of sleep pattern, the clinical signs presumably reflecting the area of CNS most affected.
- Ocular disease is not uncommon in FIV-infected cats. Diagnosis of ocular disease associated with FIV infection may require careful ophthalmic examination and is often not associated with obvious loss of vision. Anterior uveitis, glaucoma or pars planitis have all been described in FIV-infected cats, and it has been suggested that the syndrome of idiopathic uveitis seen in cats over six years old might be FIV-related.
- There is some evidence that FIV may be associated with an increased prevalence of neoplasia.
- Clinical signs in FIV infections are often associated with secondary infections.

  - Many FIV-infected cats with chronic stomatitis also have persistent feline calicivirus (FCV) infection in the oropharynx, although whether this indicates a causative role for FCV in the disease or merely increased FCV excretion by immunosuppressed cats is not known.

o Cats with chronic upper respiratory tract disease are also often infected with FCV or feline herpesvirus. In both chronic oral and chronic respiratory disease, bacterial infection undoubtedly also plays a role as antibiotic therapy can alleviate, but usually not eradicate, the clinical signs. Severe systemic herpesvirus infection has also been reported in FIV-infected cats.

o Severe systemic cowpox virus infections have been reported in FIV-infected cats.

o Active toxoplasmosis appears to be more common in FIV-infected than non-infected cats, and FIV-induced immunosuppression may be associated with clinical toxoplasmosis in cats.

o Chronic skin disease in FIV-infected cats has been associated with parasites, such as *Notoedres*, *Cheyletiella* and *Demodex* species, and with various fungal and bacterial infections.

o Other opportunist or secondary infections which may be associated with FIV infection include haemobartonellosis, intestinal coccidiosis, candidiasis, aspergillosis, cryptococcosis, and pseudomonad and mycobacterial infections.

o Co-infection of FIV and feline leukaemia virus (FeLV) may be associated with very rapid development of immunodeficiency and clinical disease both in the field and experimentally. Co-infection of FIV and FeLV is, however, uncommon because most cats with FeLV are infected when young, whereas FIV infection is more common in older cats.

o No association has been found between FIV infection and feline coronavirus infection or clinical feline infectious peritonitis

DIAGNOSIS

Antibody tests

FIV can be isolated from most cats with antibody, so antibody detection is the most frequently used method for diagnosis of FIV infection. Several ELISA and immunoconcentration kits are commercially available for detecting antibody reactive with the core p24 antigen of FIV. These assays are especially useful for the practice laboratory, and kits are available which combine tests for FIV antibody and FeLV antigen in the same kit.

Most ELISA-based tests give occasional false positive results, and large diagnostic laboratories therefore often use a further serological test for confirmation. Immunoblots, or Western blots, are most frequently used as this technique is very specific. However, even with immunoblotting, there can be some difficulty interpreting borderline reactions. Some laboratories use an immunofluorescence assay which is also claimed to be very specific. ELISAs developed in house, which test for antibody against, for example, virus-envelope antigens, are also used by some laboratories. Other techniques, such as radioimmune precipitation assays (RIPA) and virus neutralisation tests, are mainly used for research rather than diagnosis.

Interpretation of FIV serology

- All serological techniques may occasionally give apparently 'false' negative results in FIV-infected cats, and most ELISA-based tests give occasional false positives.
- Although most cats produce antibody within a few weeks of FIV infection, some cats can remain seronegative for up to a year.
- Furthermore, some severely ill cats may have little or no detectable antibody – a similar phenomenon is sometimes seen in terminal AIDS in man, and may be due to large amounts of virus antigen binding all the antibody or to profound immunosuppression.
- Detection of antibody should be interpreted with care, and in the context of the clinical reason for testing.
- In a healthy cat, antibody detection cannot be used to make a reliable prognosis as the incubation period to disease may be many years, and it may be that some cats never become clinically ill. However, field surveys suggest that many cats do eventually progress to AIDS.
- Therefore, detection of virus or antibody in an ill cat may be irrelevant to the current disease.

Virus isolation

Virus isolation is expensive and time consuming, and, as most cats with antibody are also viraemic, laboratory diagnosis of infection is generally by antibody detection. Occasionally, however, virus isolation may be necessary to demonstrate infection, for example in very recently infected cats or terminally ill cats with no detectable antibody.

One or more millilitres of blood are collected in heparin and immediately diluted with cell culture or transport medium. Lymphocytes and monocytes are isolated by centrifugation, and incubated in culture medium, initially with a mitogen of cat T-cells, concanavalin A (con A), to stimulate the lymphocytes to divide. After 2–3 days, the cells are washed and resuspended in culture medium as before, but without con A, and usually with interleukin 2 added. Fresh, stimulated, uninfected lymphocytes and media are added every 10 days or so, and the culture is tested for FIV production approximately every week for 6 or more weeks by looking for cytopathic effects, by electron microscopy or by assays for reverse transcriptase or virus antigen production.

Other detection methods, such as polymerase chain reaction and antigen ELISAs, are used experimentally but are not generally available commercially.

Other laboratory investigations

Other laboratory investigations which might corroborate a diagnosis of FIV-related disease include:

- persistent leucopenia, especially lymphopenia and neutropenia;
- anaemia;
- hypergammaglobulinaemia.

Lymph node biopsy may reveal follicular hyperplasia, or atrophy and involution.

In the future, measurement of circulating CD4 cell numbers and CD4:CD8 ratios may be more routinely available to aid diagnosis of immunosuppression, although even these can be difficult to correlate with clinical immuno-suppression.

PATHOGENESIS (Figure 5.1)

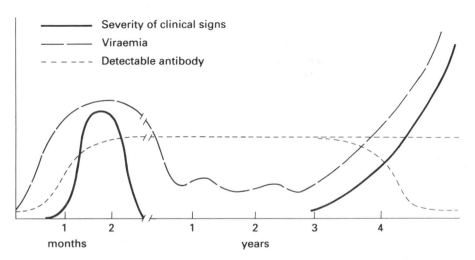

Severity of clinical signs
Viraemia
Detectable antibody

months   years

Figure 5.1 Diagram showing the probable pathogenesis of FIV infection

- Pathogenesis of FIV is not fully understood.
- Virus is isolated from blood, lymphoid organs, saliva and cerebrospinal fluid, and can be grown *in vitro* in lymphocytes, macrophages and astrocytes.
- Some strains of FIV can also grow in other cell types, for example in some feline fibroblast cell lines.
- Cats can be experimentally infected by subcutaneous, intramuscular, intra-peritoneal or intravenous inoculation.
- After experimental inoculation of kittens with high doses of FIV, virus can be isolated from lymphocytes at 1 week, and antibody detected after about 3 weeks, but time to viraemia and seroconversion is much longer if inoculated with smaller doses of virus.
- Lymphadenopathy is usually seen after 4–6 weeks experimentally, but severity depends on the dose and strain of virus, and on the age of cats when inoculated.
- Acute lymphadenopathy may be accompanied by mild pyrexia and leuco-penia, including lymphopenia and neutropenia.

- The lymphadenopathy usually disappears after 2–3 months.
- Cats then generally remain healthy for several years. Severe, chronic disease seen in the field has not been consistently reproduced experimentally. Field studies suggest clinically asymptomatic infection may last at least 3–5 years.
- Not yet known what triggers the onset of terminal AIDS-like disease in cats.
- Deficiencies in some immune functions can be detected within a few months of infection and more profound immune dysfunction gradually develops with time.

  - Decreased numbers of circulating CD4 cells and ratios of CD4:CD8 cells.
  - Reduced *in vitro* proliferation responses to some mitogens and *in vivo* responses to some antigens can be detected within the first 10 months after infection.
  - FIV causes a transient decreased expression of CD4 antigen and syncytium formation in CD4 cell cultures.
  - Persistent infection causes a progressive decreased expression of major histocompatibility complex type II antigens (MHCII).

Theories of how feline AIDS develops include:

- AIDS-like disease develops when the number of functional CD4 cells falls below a critical level due to overwhelming infection of lymphoreticular system.
- CD4 cell developmental disturbance caused by infection of macrophages and other antigen-presenting cells.
- Virus is constantly mutating in order to escape the cat's immune response, and AIDS occurs when the virus finally manages this.
- FIV infection may cause autoimmune responses against the cat's own immune system.
- Secondary infections may cause clinical AIDS either by causing mild immuno-suppression themselves or by stimulating lymphocyte multiplication and macrophage activation, thereby enhancing FIV replication in these cells.
- Some pathogens, e.g. felid herpesvirus-1, may directly enhance FIV replication.

Neurological disease is thought usually to be caused directly by FIV replication in the CNS.

TREATMENT

Treatment is largely a matter of controlling secondary infections and alleviating clinical signs.

- Antibiotics are often used to control secondary and opportunist bacterial infections.
- Surgery may temporarily alleviate chronic stomatitis and gingivitis in some cats.
- Corticosteroids or megoestrol acetate may also help moderate systemic signs but probably have little long-term beneficial effect.

Antiviral therapy

Some of the drugs being developed or used to treat HIV also inhibit FIV in cell culture and some clinical effect has been claimed for 9-(2-phosphonomethoxyethyl)adenine (PMEA) and 3'-azido-3'deoxythymidine (AZT; zidovudine) in cats. In experimental studies, PMEA has been shown to inhibit detectable FIV infection if given before virus inoculation, although viraemia developed once treatment stopped. In similar experiments, AZT in very high doses delayed but did not prevent detectable FIV infection. Some preliminary work suggests that PMEA and AZT might enable clinical recovery in some field cases (but without elimination of virus infection). In the authors' experience, treatment of field cases with AZT has generally been disappointing although a few cats did show temporary clinical improvement within a few weeks of the onset of treatment. AZT can have quite severe side effects in cats, including anaemia and liver damage, particularly at high doses or after prolonged treatment.

PREVENTION AND CONTROL

Currently no vaccine is available, therefore control of FIV infection relies on avoiding cat-to-cat transmission.

- In pet cats kept alone or in small groups, the best if not the easiest way to reduce risk of infection is prevention of roaming and fighting.
- There is no evidence that neutering reduces risk of infection in males.
- If either the new cat or any existing cats are infected with FIV, new cats ought not to be introduced into a household as this will lead to fighting and increased risk of transmission.
- However, in a stable multi-cat household in which fighting is rare, the risk of transmission from infected to non-infected cats may be small.
- There is no humane reason why a cat should be killed simply because it is infected with FIV, although it has been suggested that owners of infected cats have a moral duty to prevent their cats from roaming.
- In a breeding colony with no evidence of FIV infection, avoid the introduction of seropositive cats by antibody testing and quarantine.
- If the colony contains cats seropositive for FIV, it is probably best to separate or rehouse infected cats. Although detectable queen-to-kitten transmission is rare, it is inadvisable to breed from infected cats.

In a boarding or rescue cattery, cats ought to be housed in separate pens to avoid fighting. Infection does not appear to spread on fomites or feeding dishes, and if the recommendations for preventing spread of respiratory disease are followed, there should be no risk of FIV transmission. If cats do have to be housed together in a rescue cattery, they should be quarantined for, say, 12 weeks on entering the cattery, then tested for FIV antibody before being allowed to mix with other FIV-negative cats.

6   FELINE COWPOX

AETIOLOGY

Cowpox virus is member of the orthopoxvirus group in the family Poxviridae. Other orthopoxviruses include smallpox virus, now eradicated, vaccinia virus (the modern smallpox vaccine), infectious ectromelia virus of mice, monkeypox and camelpox viruses, and raccoonpox and California volepox viruses.

All the orthopoxviruses are very closely related and antigenically extremely similar. However, each can be identified by a combination of biological tests, minor serological differences and genome analysis.

The orthopoxviruses must not be confused with the parapoxviruses such as pseudocowpox and orf viruses. Although both genera are members of the family Poxviridae, each genus has a different morphology of the virus particle and there is no useful immunological relationship between the two.

EPIDEMIOLOGY

Cowpox virus is only found in Eurasia. Most reports of cowpox virus elsewhere in the world refer to vaccinia virus (the smallpox vaccine) which, when human vaccination was widespread, occasionally escaped into domestic livestock.

Cowpox virus has a very wide host range which includes cattle, man, domestic cats and various zoo animals (Figure 6.1). However, the reservoir host is wild rodents. Antibody to cowpox virus is found in wild voles and woodmice in Western Europe, and virus has been isolated from other rodents in Eastern Europe and Eurasia.

Bovine cowpox is very rare (unlike infection with pseudocowpox virus which is enzootic in cattle world-wide.) Cowpox virus causes teat lesions in cattle, and may spread rapidly through the herd on milking equipment. Cattle-to-man transmission can occur, but most people with cowpox have had no contact with cattle.

The most commonly recognised host of cowpox virus is the domestic cat. About one-half of human cases in the UK can be traced to contact with an infected cat.

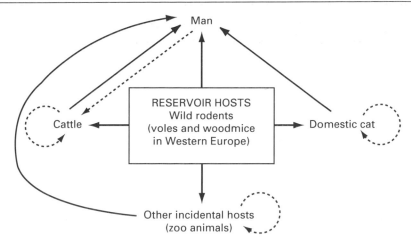

Figure 6.1 Probable epidemiology of cowpox

- Cats probably become infected when hunting.
- Most affected cats are adult and come from rural environments, and almost all are known by their owners to hunt small mammals.
- Most feline cases are seen in the autumn (Figure 6.2), probably because small mammal populations are at their maximum size and because individual rodents are most active and therefore are most prone to capture at that time of year.

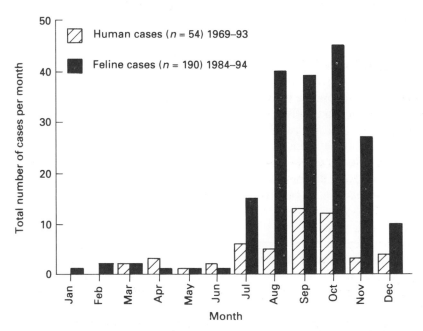

Figure 6.2 Graph showing markedly increased incidence of cowpox in both cats and man in the autumn

- Cat-to-cat transmission can occur, but generally causes only asymptomatic infection in the recipient cat.

    Cowpox virus has also been isolated from exotic cats, including cheetahs, lions, pumas, ocelots and lynx in European zoos, and also from okapi, elephants, rhinoceroses, and anteaters.

CLINICAL SIGNS

- Usually first presented for veterinary attention with widespread skin lesions.
- Further examination may reveal that cat originally had a single skin lesion, usually on the head, neck or a forelimb. These primary lesions vary in character from large abscesses or areas of cellulitis to small, scabbed papules or rodent-ulcer-like lesions. However, many owners describe primary lesions as having developed from a small, bite-like wound.
- The widespread secondary skin lesions develop a few days to weeks (average 10 days) after primary lesion is first noticed. Secondary lesions first appear as small, randomly distributed erythematous nodules, which over 3–5 days develop into ulcerated papules up to 1 cm diameter. These quickly become scabbed.
- The lesions are often not pruritic, but may be if secondarily infected or when healing.
- The scabs dry and separate after a further 2–3 weeks. New hair soon grows, and most cats are completely recovered in 6–8 weeks.
- Approximately one in five cats may also develop a mild, serous nasal discharge, conjunctivitis or transient diarrhoea, and some cats may be depressed and anorexic.
- More severe or chronic systemic signs, or delayed healing of skin lesions, may result from secondary bacterial infection, especially of the primary lesion, or immunodeficiency either from corticosteroid treatment, severe concurrent disease (e.g. chronic renal failure) or infection with feline leukaemia virus or feline immunodeficiency virus.
- Severe systemic signs, particularly evidence of pneumonia or in conjunction with underlying immunosuppressive disease, suggest a poor prognosis, and euthanasia might be considered.

Cowpox in exotic and big cats

- Cowpox is often a more severe disease in non-domestic cats.
- Infected cheetahs often develop pneumonia and may die before any skin lesions develop.
- High mortality in animals infected with cowpox virus has also been reported in lions, ocelots and lynx.

DIAGNOSIS

Clinical signs

With experience, many veterinary surgeons can accurately diagnose most cases of cowpox in cats on clinical signs alone. Differential diagnoses might include cat bite abscesses, neoplasia, eosinophilic granuloma, and miliary eczema, although the discrete, widespread lesions of cowpox are quite characteristic.

Fixed biopsy material

This can be examined microscopically for the characteristic eosinophilic intra-cytoplasmic inclusion bodies of cowpox virus. However, these are not always easily found, and immunostaining may be necessary for confirmation.

Virus isolation

Isolation can be attempted on dry unfixed scab material. This can be sent by mail without the need for special transport medium. Electron microscopy of scab material enables rapid diagnosis in three out of four cases, but virus isolation is more sensitive. However, isolation may take up to 10 days.

Serum

Serum can be tested for antibody using several assays. An immuno-fluorescence (IF) test is now routinely used as it is both sensitive and relatively rapid. Because cowpox virus is not enzootic in cats, detection of antibody is almost diagnostic of present infection. However, using class-specific mono-clonal antibodies, the IF test can be modified to detect only IgM, indicative of present infection.

TREATMENT AND PREVENTION

There is no specific treatment for cowpox, so treatment usually consists of broad-spectrum antibiotics to control secondary and concurrent bacterial infection. Large lesions may be cleaned with antiseptics, and an Elizabethan collar or paw-bandaging may be necessary to prevent scratching.

Corticosteroids should be avoided as they may exacerbate the condition.

There is no vaccine available, and feline cowpox is not common enough to warrant development of one.

Control in exotic and big cats

Vaccinia virus does not grow well in cats, and when tested did not provoke an antibody response in a cheetah. Control of disease in exotic cat collections therefore relies largely on prompt diagnosis and isolation of affected individuals.

PUBLIC HEALTH ASPECTS

- Cats are the source of about half of all human cowpox virus infections.
- Human infection is often limited to a single lesion on the hand or face, but spread to other sites may occur, for example hand to face.
- Widespread infection and severe disease can develop in immunosuppressed individuals or those with a pre-existing skin disease. Human cowpox often also causes some systemic illness with 'flu-like symptoms, and may require hospitalisation.
- Occasional human deaths have also been reported.
- Smallpox vaccination, even recent, may not provide complete protection against primary cowpox virus infection, although it might prevent the development of more severe disease.

Human cowpox is not common: two or three cases are reported each year in the UK. Experience suggests that transmission from cats to humans is unlikely if basic hygiene precautions are taken.

Veterinary surgeons and others handling infected cats should wear gloves and take care not to allow infected material into wounds or the eyes. Young children, the elderly and those with a pre-existing skin condition or with debilitative or immunosuppressive disease should avoid contact with the cat while the scabs remain.

The virus is extremely hardy, and may remain infectious in dry material kept cool for several months or even years. However, it is susceptible to most disinfectants, particularly hypochlorite.

7 FELINE SPONGIFORM ENCEPHALOPATHY

AETIOLOGY

Little is known specifically about the agent of FSE. Indeed the nature of the infectious agents causing infectious spongiform encephalopathies in other species (e.g. scrapie in sheep, bovine spongiform encephalopathy (BSE) in cattle, and Creutzfeld–Jacob disease and kuru in man) is also not well understood.

Theories as to their structure include either a protein ('prion') or a protein–nucleic acid ('virino') combination. Scrapie infectivity is associated with protein fibrils (scrapie associated fibrils (SAF)), in which it has not been possible to detect a scrapie-specific nucleic acid. The spongiform encephalopathy agents are extremely hardy: they will survive extremely high temperatures and UV-irradiation which would normally destroy nucleic acids. However, it is possible that the protein component is in some way able to protect a very small nucleic acid (possibly RNA) genome, and small pieces of protected cellular RNA have been found bound up in SAF. In addition, no other replicating 'life-form' is known which does not contain nucleic acid, and it is difficult to conceive how a protein could transmit so much strain-specific variation (strains can be typed by comparison of their pathogenicity in laboratory mice) as is found among different scrapie strains. On the other hand, the protein fibrils associated with the spongiform encephalopathies are encoded by genes found in normal tissues, and the fibrils themselves appear to consist of a host cell protein (PrP) which has been abnormally processed (modified PrP) during infection. One suggestion is that the infectious agent is simply abnormally folded protein (prion) which somehow catalyses (crystallises?) the abnormal folding of otherwise normal protein produced in CNS and other tissues, thereby giving the impression of replication.

PATHOGENESIS

- The routes of infection in cats are not known, although in other species ingestion, transplacental spread and skin inoculation can all occur.
- The most likely route of feline infection is probably oral, with food as the most likely source of FSE agent.
- The time between inoculation and the development of disease in cats is not yet known, nor is it known what tissues other than CNS the infectious agent may be found in. It is not known if transplacental or other routes of cat-to-cat transmission can occur.

EPIDEMIOLOGY

FSE is not common, and has so far only been reported in cats either in or originating from Britain. Most cases (over 60) have been reported in domestic cats, but several cases of FSE have also been documented in non-domestic cats; (pumas, cheetahs and an ocelot) in zoological collections.

Retrospective surveys of feline CNS material taken at necropsy suggest that FSE is a relatively new disease of cats. The first cases were reported in 1990, soon after the emergence of BSE in cattle.

Domestic cats that developed FSE have been fed a broad range of different proprietary cat foods and table scraps during their lifetime, so it is difficult to pinpoint the source of infection. One might, however, speculate that FSE has developed in domestic cats through exposure to BSE or a BSE-like agent.

At the time of writing, there are no published results available from attempts to produce experimental infections in cats using material from cattle with BSE. However, recent experiments aimed at typing BSE and FSE by mouse pathogenesis studies have shown that BSE is different from known scrapie strains but that BSE and FSE are indistinguishable.

CLINICAL SIGNS

- Ataxia and incoordination
- Hyperaesthesia
- Hypermetria
- Hypersalivation
- Muscle tremors
- Changes in behaviour.

DIAGNOSIS

Diagnosis can only be made post mortem.

Diagnosis is by the demonstration of characteristic histopathology of the brain at necropsy, and by demonstration of fibrils in CNS tissue by electron microscopy, and of modified PrP by immunostaining.

PUBLIC HEALTH ASPECTS

The risk of human infection from affected cats is not known, as the identity of the causative agent and its relationship to the causes of spongiform encephalopathy in other species are not known. Even if the agent is infectious to man, it is highly unlikely that a live cat could be a source of human infection. However, it would be prudent to handle all tissues taken post mortem from suspect cases with extreme care.

FSE is a notifiable disease in the UK.

Section 2
MAJOR CANINE INFECTIOUS DISEASES

SECTION 2

8 CANINE INFECTIOUS GASTROENTERITIS

There are many causes of infectious enteritis in the dog. Canine parvovirus (CPV) and canine distemper virus (CDV) (see Chapter 10) are responsible for the more severe and acute manifestations whereas canine coronavirus (CCV), canine rotavirus (CRV), *Campylobacter* spp, *Salmonella* spp and clostridia are usually associated with milder disease. Other agents (e.g. caliciviruses, a herpesvirus and enteroviruses; see Section 3) have also been described in the faeces of dogs with diarrhoea, and it is possible that some of these may be responsible for some cases of enteritis.

AETIOLOGY

Canine parvovirus (CPV)

- Two unrelated parvoviruses can infect dogs: CPV-1 or the minute virus of canines, and CPV-2.
- Parvoviruses are non-enveloped particles of approximately 18–26 nm in diameter.
- CPV-2 is very closely related to feline panleucopenia virus (FPV) (see Chapter 2).
- But CPV-1 and CPV-2 only appear to infect members of the Canidae family.
- CPV-2 is extremely stable in the external environment (up to 5 months in faecal material under favourable conditions).
- CPV-1 and CPV-2 are resistant to most common disinfectants but are destroyed by formalin, glutaraldehyde and chlorine compounds.

Canine coronavirus (CCV)

- Typical coronavirus containing single stranded RNA and three structural proteins.
- The peplomer or spike proteins project from the envelope of the virus and are responsible for the virus's characteristic crown or 'corona' of large petals from which it gets its name.

- CCV is very closely related to feline coronavirus (see Chapter 3) and is infectious to dogs, cats and pigs.
- There is slight variation in pathogenicity between isolates.
- One serotype only, although minor antigenic differences between isolates exist.
- Coronavirus infectivity is reduced or eliminated by detergents which destroy the lipid envelope.
- CCV is labile in the external environment (it may survive up to 48 hours in faecal material depending upon the ambient temperature).

Canine rotavirus (CRV)

- CRV is a typical rotavirus, consisting of a double-stranded RNA genome within a non-enveloped double-layered capsid approximately 70 nm in diameter.
- CRV is stable in the external environment; rotaviruses retain their infectivity at pH 3 and are insensitive to many detergents, but are readily destroyed by formalin, glutaraldehyde and chlorine compounds.

Campylobacter spp

- Gram-negative, slender, curved rod (1.5–5 μm by 0.2–0.5 μm) which may be curve-, S- or gull-shaped, found singly, in pairs or in chains.
- *C. jejuni* is the organism usually associated with diarrhoea in the dog although *C. coli* may be isolated on occasions.

See also salmonellosis (Chapter 40) and colibacillosis (Chapter 39).

PATHOGENESIS AND PATHOLOGY

CPV infection

CPV-2 is a far more important pathogen than CPV-1, and a common cause of disease in dogs of all ages and breeds. CPV-1 has been demonstrated in faeces of dogs with mild diarrhoea but its pathogenicity is unclear.

The primary route of natural CPV-2 infection is by ingestion, although transplacental transmission can also occur. CPV-2 requires actively dividing cells to replicate, and thus it has a predilection for the cells of the lymphoid system, bone marrow and crypt epithelia of the intestinal tract, and, in puppies under 4 weeks of age, cardiac myocytes.

After ingestion, CPV-2 initially replicates in oropharyngeal, mesenteric and thymic lymphoid tissue. Subsequent haematogenous generalisation distributes the virus to lymphoid tissue, bone marrow, intestinal epithelial cells, lungs, liver and kidney. Infection of these tissues leads to the development of clinical signs from day 4 post-infection.

Virus particles may be found in faeces as early as day 3 after inoculation, increasing in number up to day 6, then declining markedly by day 12. CPV-2 is rarely found in faecal material as virus shedding ceases once clinical signs develop.

CPV-2 cardiomyopathy only occurs if pups are infected in the first 4 weeks of life and the pups have no maternally derived antibody.

Pathological findings of CPV-2 intestinal infection

Gross
Thickening of intestinal walls as a result of subserosal congestion and the presence of watery, often haemorrhagic contents. Mesenteric lymph nodes may be enlarged and oedematous. Thymic atrophy may be present.

Histopathology
Changes may be seen either throughout the small intestine or in restricted areas. They arise from destruction of epithelial cells lining crypts and an inability to replace the normal turnover of intestinal epithelium. Disruption of the villous architecture is characterised by blunting and fusing of villi, and the presence of an immature, flattened epithelium. Intranuclear inclusion bodies may be seen in the early stages of infection. Necrosis and depletion of lymphoid tissue may also occur. An inflammatory response develops as a result of secondary bacterial infection.

Pathological findings of CPV-2 myocardial infection

Gross
Signs of congestive heart failure; such as pulmonary oedema, hepatic congestion, a dilated flaccid heart, ascites and hydrothorax may be evident. Cardiac muscle may contain pale white streaks associated with myocardial necrosis and cellular infiltrates.

Histopathology
CPV-2 infection is characterised by a non-suppurative cardiomyopathy. In the early stages degeneration and loss of cardiac myocytes without an inflammatory cell infiltration is evident. By day 52 a lymphocytic infiltration and fibrosis may be present. Intranuclear inclusion bodies are frequent.

CCV infection

Dogs of all ages and breeds appear to be susceptible to CCV infection. The natural route of infection is thought to be primarily by ingestion, although it is possible to infect dogs intranasally. After ingestion, CCV infects the mucosal epithelium overlying the upper two-thirds of small intestinal villi and, to a lesser extent, the colonic mucosa.

Viraemia has not been demonstrated but virus has also been isolated from liver, meninges, lung and mesenteric and peripheral lymph nodes after oral inoculation. The clinical significance of such spread is not known.

Virus is shed in faeces from day 3 to 16 post-inoculation, and virus neutralising antibodies are detectable in serum from days 7 to 10.

Pathological findings of CCV infection

Gross
Distension of intestinal loops by watery digesta and enlarged oedematous mesenteric lymph nodes.

Histopathology
Lesions are restricted to atrophy and fusion of intestinal villi and deepening of crypts, increased cellularity of the lamina propria and flattening of epithelial cells. Discharge of goblet cells may be evident and probably reflects partial healing after the earlier more severe damage. Histological evidence of recovery of the intestinal mucosa may be evident from day seven onwards.

CRV infection

Canine rotavirus has been isolated from both clinically normal young dogs and from dogs with diarrhoea. The natural route of infection is probably by ingestion of virus particles. Infection is limited to the gastrointestinal tract, and it is difficult to experimentally infect dogs over 6 months of age. Rotaviruses infect the villous epithelial cells on the upper one-half to one-third of the villi in jejunum and ileum, and histopathological changes are limited to mild or moderate villous atrophy.

Campylobacteriosis

The reported incidence of *Campylobacter* spp in dogs with or without diarrhoea varies considerably, and many dogs are asymptomatic carriers. Thus the significance of *Campylobacter* spp as a cause of gastrointestinal disease in dogs is not clear. The severity of disease is probably dependent upon the number of organisms present, their ability to produce various toxins, previous exposure to *Campylobacter* spp, the presence of other enteric pathogens and the development of protective antibody. In general campylobacteriosis causes only mild disease, and experimental infections are usually less severe than field infections suggesting that other factors or organisms may play a role in its pathogenesis.

Pathological findings of campylobacteriosis

Gross
Fluid colonic contents and thickening, congestion and oedema of the colonic mucosa.

Histopathology
Decrease in enterocyte height and numbers of goblet cells, and hyperplasia of epithelial glands. Villus height may be reduced. Subepithelial congestion, haemorrhage and inflammation may be evident.

CLINICAL SIGNS

CPV-2 infection

The severity of enteric disease caused by canine parvovirus is very variable. Many natural infections appear to be subclinical, and severe disease is difficult to reproduce experimentally. However, CPV-2 has been reported to account for between 25% and 50% of acute diarrhoea cases in dogs.

The diarrhoea results from loss of absorptive and digestive capacities but an inflammatory response may contribute a secretory component if a secondary bacterial infection occurs.

Mortality rates may be as high as 7–10% in pups but in adults they are generally less than 1%, although in an outbreak at one rescue kennel, 92% of stray dogs older than eight months of age were reported to die of CPV-2 enteropathy.

Clinical features include:

- Incubation period of 4–7 days.
- Initially see acute onset, protracted and severe vomiting with depression and anorexia.
- Watery often haemorrhagic diarrhoea developing 6–24 hours later.
- Pyrexia is common.
- Haematological investigation may show a lymphopenia, associated with viral infection of lymphoid tissue, and an increased packed cell volume as a result of dehydration.
- Weight loss may be dramatic.
- Death may occur within 72 hours of the onset of clinical signs.

Myocardial disease associated with CPV-2 infection is no longer at all common as most pups are protected during the first few weeks of life by maternally derived antibody.

Clinical features reported with myocardial CPV-2 infection include:

- Clinical signs of myocardial disease develop 3–7 weeks after CPV-2 infection.
- Death in up to 70% of affected pups by 8 weeks of age. Of the remaining 30%, many will die some months or years later of acute or chronic cardiac failure.
- Most affected pups collapse and die rapidly within minutes of acute cardiac failure.
- Premonitory signs are not often observed, but on occasions dyspnoea, crying and retching have been recorded.

CCV infection

CCV infection generally causes only a mild diarrhoea, and older dogs often show no clinical signs. Younger dogs, up to 12 weeks of age, appear to show a greater susceptibility to the more severe forms of the disease.

Clinical features include:

- Incubation period of 1–5 days.
- Vomiting and diarrhoea are the predominant clinical signs.
- Depression, anorexia and lethargy may be a feature in some cases.
- Faeces vary from a cowpat-like consistency to watery. On occasions the diarrhoea may be haemorrhagic.
- Pyrexia and leucopenia are not features of CCV infection.
- Spontaneous recovery usually occurs 7–10 days after the onset of clinical signs, but diarrhoea may persist for up to 4 weeks.

CRV infection

CRV infection is probably most significant in young puppies where it may cause diarrhoea between 1 and 6 days post-infection.

- Watery diarrhoea is the predominant clinical feature.
- Depression, lethargy and inappetance.
- Vomiting, haemorrhagic diarrhoea, pyrexia and leucopenia are not generally features of CRV infection.
- Spontaneous recovery will usually occur within 7 days if supportive treatment is given.

Campylobacteriosis

Dogs less than 6 months of age are usually the most severely affected. Stress associated with illness or hospitalisation may increase an animal's susceptibility to infection.

- The diarrhoea usually varies from a cowpat-like consistency to watery.
- Blood and mucus may be present.
- Diarrhoea is usually self-limiting but occasionally it may persist for several months.
- Inappetance, occasional vomiting and pyrexia may also be seen.

DIAGNOSIS

A presumptive diagnosis of viral gastroenteritis may be made on the basis of the clinical signs and/or histopathology, especially if immunocytochemical staining is used. Vomiting and diarrhoea with severe leucopenia early in the disease and characteristic post-mortem findings may strongly suggest CPV-2 infection. However, because of the lack of distinctive clinical or pathological features in many cases, a definitive diagnosis can only be made if the infectious agents are detected and identified.

Virus detection and isolation

For isolation of CCV or parvovirus in cell culture, fresh faecal material should be placed in virus transport medium and submitted immediately by first class post to a specialist laboratory. Faecal samples must be collected as soon as possible after the onset of clinical signs.

While some viruses grow rapidly from some samples, it may take several weeks before a formal laboratory result is obtained for attempted isolation.

Remember that CPV can be difficult to detect in faeces once clinical signs have developed, and that CCV is labile and so samples must arrive at the laboratory quickly.

Faecal samples can also be examined by electron microscopy for virus particles. This technique is especially useful for rotavirus which can be difficult to grow in cell culture. Immunoconcentration may be a useful technique for the detection of parvovirus.

CPV can also be detected in faeces by haemagglutination or by using commercially available antigen-detection kits. The CPV antigen-capture CITE assay marketed by Iddex Corp. appears to be both sensitive and specific compared with haemagglutination and isolation, and can also detect feline parvovirus in faeces from some cases of feline panleucopenia.

Virus serology

Serology is of limited value in CPV-2 infection as a significant rise in antibody titre during the course of clinical disease may not occur. CPV-2-infected dogs may already have developed high antibody titres by 7 days after inoculation and prior to onset of clinical signs. Furthermore, the development of CPV-2 disease often occurs around the same time as vaccination, so even rises in antibody titre can be difficult to interpret. However, estimation of Ig M titres to CPV-2 may be useful for demonstrating some acute infections.

Serology may be of more use for the retrospective diagnosis of CCV infection, particularly in non-vaccinated populations. Virus neutralising (VN) antibodies to CCV first appear 7 days after inoculation and continue to rise over subsequent weeks. A serum sample should be obtained at the onset of clinical signs and again 2 weeks later. VN antibodies may also be epidemiologically useful as they can be used to differentiate different strains of CCV.

Diagnosis of campylobacteriosis

- *Campylobacter* spp organisms may survive for up to 3 days in faecal material.
- However, fresh faecal samples should be examined at the earliest possible opportunity in order to increase the possibility of making a definitive diagnosis.
- *C. jejuni* may be visualised using either dark-field or phase-contrast light microscopy.
- Isolation may also be attempted on blood-agar plates in an oxygen-reduced atmosphere.

TREATMENT

- There are no antiviral drugs available to treat viral gastroenteritis.
- Supportive treatment is required for the more serious cases.

Fluid therapy

Fluid and electrolyte loss can be managed through the administration of crystalloids parenterally. Lactated Ringer's solution is preferred where significant vomiting and diarrhoea are present. The fluid should be administered through an intravenous catheter at a rate of 100–150 ml/kg/day until the patient is rehydrated and then at a rate of 66 ml/kg/day for maintenance plus an amount to cover any extraordinary losses (vomiting or diarrhoea).

Antiemetics

Antiemetic therapy with metoclopromide (0.2–0.5 mg/kg orally or by subcutaneous injection every 6–8 hours, or 1–2 mg/kg IV over 24 hours as a slow infusion).

Antibiotics

Antibiotic therapy is not indicated for CCV or CRV infection unless significant melaena is present. However, systemic antibiotic use is recommended for CPV-2 infections where significant damage to the gastrointestinal mucosa is present.

Appropriate antibiotics include:

- Amoxycillin/clavulanate (8.75 mg/kg IM or subcutaneous daily, or 12–25 mg/kg orally twice daily) or a potentiated sulphonamide.
- Erythromycin is the drug of choice to treat campylobacteriosis (10 mg/kg orally, three times daily).

Diet

Water only should be made available for 48 hours.

Once the vomiting has subsided, feed a bland, highly digestible diet (e.g. a commercial 'clinical' convalescent diet, rice and chicken, or cottage cheese) for 7–10 days.

EPIDEMIOLOGY

CPV-2

CPV-2 first appeared as a cause of a severe canine enteropathy and cardiomyopathy in 1978. Its origin is not clear. The original strain of CPV-2 has now been replaced worldwide by antigenic variants CPV-2a and/or CPV-2b.

- The virus has a world-wide distribution.
- Seroprevalence rates range from 25% for family-owned dogs to 90% for kennel dogs.
- CPV-2 is extremely hardy, and can survive in the environment for more than 6 months at room temperature, and thus may be transported over long distances by fomites.
- The main source of infection is faeces from infected dogs.
- Persistent or periodic faecal shedding from infected dogs does not appear to be a feature of CPV-2 infection because of the strong immune response mounted by infected dogs.
- Neither aerosol nor transplacental infection are thought to be important.

CCV

- World-wide distribution.
- Capable of causing widespread epizootics.
- Seroprevalence rates 0–54% of pet dogs and 0–80% of kennelled dogs.
- Can also infect dogs, coyotes, cats and pigs.
- Transmission is faeco-oral, but CCV infectivity in faeces decreases rapidly over 48 hours.
- It is not known if CCV carrier states occur.
- Reinfection common – pre-existing immunity generally does not provide good protection against subsequent infection.

CRV

- Serological surveys suggest that most dogs have been infected with CRV at some time.
- Transmission occurs by direct contact with infected faeces.

Campylobacteriosis

In one report *C. jejuni* was isolated from 29% of dogs with diarrhoea compared with 4% of dogs without, but in other studies the isolation of *C. jejuni* from diarrhoeic and non-diarrhoeic dogs has been generally similar. Higher isolation rates have been reported from kennel dogs than from pet dogs.

- Younger animals are at greater risk of infection probably due to lack of previous exposure.
- Spread is via the faeco-oral route.
- Sources of the organism include faeces and contaminated meat products, particularly of poultry and wild birds, and unpasteurised milk.
- Nosocomial infections are possible.

Although canine campylobacteriosis can be zoonotic, infection of dogs and humans from a shared source is probably more common than dog-to-human transmission.

PREVENTION AND CONTROL

Canine parvovirus vaccination

When CPV first appeared in the late 1970s, modified live or inactivated feline panleucopenia vaccines were used. These induced variable protection to CPV-2 infection, generally of short duration, and only vaccines derived from CPV are now generally used.

- Inactivated CPV-2 vaccines provide protection from infection for up to one year.
- Live attenuated vaccines generally induce a longer lasting protection (up to two years' duration) and a more consistent response.

Note: Most live parvovirus vaccines of cats and dogs are shed in faeces. The degree of attenuation determines the extent of replication in and shedding of the vaccine virus from the host. A viraemia may be present 2 days post-vaccination in dogs, with antibodies appearing a day later.

- Puppies are usually vaccinated at 8 or 9 and 12 weeks old.
- Maternally derived antibody (MDA) can sometimes prevent an effective response to vaccination, but most modern live CPV vaccines are able to overcome MDA.

Maternally derived antibody and CPV vaccination

Most puppies are susceptible to field infection between 8 and 12 weeks of age. However, some puppies may be susceptible earlier and others may have MDA levels in excess of 1/40 after 12 weeks of age. The timing of vaccination will depend on the risk to the pups of field infection and their antibody titres. In general, if the risk is low, puppies need to be vaccinated with a live attenuated vaccine at 8 and 12 weeks only. If the risk of infection is great, repeated vaccination every 2–4 weeks from 6 to 12 weeks of age will protect more puppies. For many years extra doses of vaccine (at 16 weeks of age and 6 months old) were routinely given to circumvent blocking of vaccination by the large amount of MDA to CPV acquired by pups. Anecdotal evidence suggested that certain breeds of dog were predisposed to high levels of MDA in pups but larger scale surveys found no evidence to support this. However, further vaccination after 12 weeks of age is not required with most modern attenuated CPV-2 vaccines which are able to overcome high MDA titres.

Serology, in particular measurement of haemagglutination-inhibiting (HI) antibodies, can indicate whether or not puppies are susceptible to infection and vaccination. HI titres below 1/40 do not usually affect the response to live attenuated vaccines, and a single vaccination may be all that is required. However, if titres of >1/40 exist, a multiple vaccination programme may be required.

- Booster vaccines should be administered yearly.

CCV vaccination

Systemic inoculation of both live and killed CCV vaccines induces the development of serum virus neutralising antibody. Such vaccines generally do not appear to provide much protection against infection, but protection against disease is difficult to assess as experimentally inoculated dogs seldom develop significant clinical disease.

- No vaccines are available in the UK.
- Inactivated vaccines are available in some parts of Europe and the USA.
- A live vaccine sold in the USA was withdrawn following reports of a pancreatitis/meningitis syndrome associated with its use, although the precise cause of this syndrome was not determined.
- Other live attenuated vaccines have been recently developed and these may provide better protection against both infection and disease than inactivated vaccines.

Other control measures

- The prevention of infectious enteritis depends on the isolation of susceptible dogs from infected dogs and from infected material.
- Use chlorine solutions (1 in 30 dilution), formalin (1% solution), glutaraldehyde-based or other specialist disinfectants to disinfect kennels, runs, feed bowls, cleaning implements, personnel and other fomites.

Note: Most disinfectants cannot penetrate, or are inactivated by, large lumps of organic matter, so cleanliness is an essential prerequisite of disinfection.

● For breeding kennels quarantine all incoming dogs for 4 weeks.

Control of CPV-2 infection

This is very difficult, as CPV is extremely hardy in the environment. In kennels with enzootic CPV-2 infection, control is aimed at weaning puppies in isolation and vaccinating them every 2 weeks from 4 or 5 weeks of age. Such puppies should be housed in thoroughly disinfected kennels and should be isolated from other dogs.

Control of CCV infection

In enzootic kennels this is probably impossible as there are likely to be large numbers of asymptomatically infected dogs. Thus, control is aimed at whelping bitches away from other dogs and maintaining the puppies in isolation until they are at least 12 weeks of age when they will be less susceptible to the more severe manifestations of CCV infection.

Control of campylobacteriosis

Because of the large numbers of asymptomatic carriers control of campylobacteriosis is difficult. Prompt isolation and treatment of affected dogs will decrease the environmental burden of the organism. The potential for human infection with *Campylobacter* spp should be kept in mind, and appropriate hygienic measures taken.

9 INFECTIOUS CANINE HEPATITIS

AETIOLOGY

- Infectious canine hepatitis (ICH) is caused by canine adenovirus-1 (CAV-1), which is found world-wide and can infect most Canidae, although some species, including the domestic dog, are more sensitive than others.
- Skunks, raccoons and some bears can also be infected.
- Antibody has also been found in man and European badgers, but this probably reflects cross-reaction with other adenoviruses.
- Virus is hardy: it can survive several weeks at room temperature.

PATHOGENESIS

Oronasal infection is followed by replication in tonsils and Peyer's patches, spread to other lymphatic tissues and viraemia. Virus then replicates in vascular endothelial cells in many organs, and in hepatocytes, endothelial cells of renal glomerulae, and the cornea and uvea.

As well as acute disease, persistent infection of the kidneys and immune complex formation can lead to glomerulonephritis. Immune complexes also may cause corneal and uveal inflammation (blue eye). Persistently infected dogs may shed virus in their urine for up to 6 months.

CLINICAL SIGNS

The clinical signs of ICH can vary enormously in severity.

- First clinical sign is pyrexia – and this may be only clinical sign.
- At other end of the clinical spectrum, some dogs may die within 24 hours of onset of pyrexia.
- Typically, signs include:
  apathy
  anorexia
  increased thirst.

- Vomiting and diarrhoea and abdominal tenderness are also common.
- Sometimes conjunctivitis and photophobia.
- Often vascular endothelial damage leads to petechial haemorrhage on mucous membranes and sometimes skin.
- Possibly also jaundice.
- Can also be a cause of kennel cough (see Chapter 11).
- Rarely neurological signs due to haemorrhage in CNS.
- Blue eye, if seen, occurs 1–3 weeks after acute signs have disappeared.

DIAGNOSIS

Laboratory diagnosis is based on isolation of virus from nasal secretions, blood or urine, or affected tissues at necropsy. Microscopic examination of liver often reveals a characteristic pattern of tissue damage and intranuclear inclusion bodies in infected hepatocytes.

Acetone-fixed sections or tissue imprints can enable rapid diagnosis by immunofluorescence staining.

Affected dogs are often leucopenic and have elevated liver enzymes.

CONTROL

Control is largely based on vaccination, and has been very successful; infectious hepatitis caused by CAV-1 is unusual nowadays. Both live and inactivated vaccines are available. Live CAV-1 vaccines used to produce an unacceptable incidence of mild disease and blue eye, and live ICH vaccines now contain canine adenovirus-2 (CAV-2). CAV-2 is a cause of kennel cough (see Chapter 11), and CAV-2 vaccines induce protection against disease caused by both CAV-1 and CAV-2.

10 CANINE DISTEMPER

This highly contagious disease of dogs and other carnivores is still reasonably common despite several decades of vaccination. Clinical signs may involve the respiratory, alimentary and central nervous systems, and may vary in severity from very mild to rapidly fatal. In vaccinated or otherwise partially immune dogs, only the respiratory sign may be seen, making distemper an important part of the differential diagnosis of kennel cough (see Chapter 11).

AETIOLOGY

- Canine distemper virus (CDV) is a morbillivirus – same group as rinderpest, measles and phocine (seal) distemper viruses.
- Virus fairly unstable in environment and readily destroyed by most disinfectants.
- Only one serotype, so one vaccine can be used widely, but strains vary in tissue tropism and pathogenicity – hence variation in clinical signs (although the immune status of the dog and the dose of virus are obviously also important in determining the clinical outcome of infection).

PATHOGENESIS

Dogs are usually infected by aerosol.

Virus replicates in the tonsils and bronchial lymph nodes leading to viraemia (in macrophages) and further replication in widespread lymphoid tissues. Damage caused by this replication causes lymphopenia and immunosuppression.

Dogs may eliminate the virus at this stage, but if it is a very pathogenic strain, or if the dog is not able to make a good immune response, then the virus spreads to the epithelial surfaces of the respiratory, enteric and urogenital tracts, skin and CNS. The relative involvement of these tissues determines the clinical signs which develop.

CLINICAL SIGNS

- In a 'typical' case, the dog becomes pyrexic about 1 week after exposure and signs of generalised disease develop after several weeks. These may include:

  o serous-mucopurulent nasal and conjunctival discharges
  o coughing
  o dyspnoea
  o pneumonia
  o vomiting and diarrhoea
  o pyrexia
  o and, later, hyperkeratosis.

- After 2–4 weeks of generalised disease, the dog may appear to recover completely.
- Alternatively, signs of CNS disease may develop. Neurological disease can be acute or chronic, and often indicates a poor prognosis.
- In dogs which recover, persistent infection of the CNS can lead to 'old dog encephalitis' years later.
- Enamel hypoplasia can often be seen in recovered puppies.

But typical distemper is uncommon.

- The clinical signs of distemper are often much milder than in the so-called 'typical' case, and often the disease will affect mainly one organ system, for example:

  o the respiratory tract (in which case distemper needs to be distinguished from kennel cough, especially as secondary infection with *B. bronchiseptica* is common);
  o the alimentary tract; or
  o the CNS.

- In addition, there is some evidence that persistent CDV infection might be involved in the pathogenesis of rheumatoid arthritis in dogs.

DIAGNOSIS

Clinical history

Typically:

- young dog
- unvaccinated
- stray
- must be distinguished from kennel cough if only mild respiratory signs are seen.

Laboratory diagnosis

The virus is difficult to grow from clinical cases, and isolation is rarely used in routine cases. The best sample to take for attempted isolation from acute cases is heparinised blood from which primary lymphocyte and macrophage cells containing virus can be cultured.

Serology is generally unhelpful as so many healthy dogs have antibody (due to vaccination or previous infection) and by the time clinical signs develop the antibody titre has already peaked so there is usually no sign of a rising titre.

Some laboratories use an immunofluorescence test on acetone-fixed smears of conjunctiva, tonsil or buffy coat for diagnosis of acute cases.

A definitive diagnosis is most easily made post mortem.

- Eosinophilic inclusions can be seen in lymphoid and epithelial tissues (especially bladder and respiratory mucosa).
- Immune staining can be useful for identifying infected tissues.

TREATMENT

- There is no specific treatment, except, perhaps, antiglobulin.
- Fluid therapy for dehydration, broad-spectrum antibiotics to control secondary bacterial infections.
- Good nursing will often enable dogs to recover – but euthanasia might be recommended if CNS signs are severe or persistent.

PREVENTION

- Vaccines are modified live because killed vaccines tended not to protect very well.
- Maternal antibody has generally declined to non-interfering levels by 8–12 weeks, so puppies are generally immunised at 9 and 12 weeks or isolated and immunised at 12 weeks only.
- Following two vaccinations, some dogs can remain protected for 7 years or more – but best not to rely on this and to boost after one year and then annually or every other year.
- Vaccinated animals can still be subclinically infected and thereby a source of infection and disease to non-vaccinated dogs.

Note: The virus is labile, and therefore so is the vaccine when reconstituted with water (maximum 24 hours at 20°C in dark – much less at higher temperatures and in daylight).

- Measles virus is closely enough related to CDV that the immune response induced by measles vaccination may protect against distemper. But the two viruses are antigenically sufficiently different that measles vaccination can provoke protective immunity in the presence of maternally-derived antibody to CDV. Therefore measles vaccine can be used in puppies at risk of infection from about 6 weeks of age. However, recent studies suggest that some modern distemper vaccines may be equally or even more effective at this age.

PUBLIC HEALTH RISKS

Suspicions that canine distemper virus might be associated with multiple sclerosis in man have proved groundless. However, a possible association of distemper virus with Paget's disease in man has recently been reported.

OTHER HOSTS

Canine distemper virus can infect various wild dog species, and mustelids, particularly ferrets and possibly including Eurasian badgers.

Canine distemper virus can also infect cats. In domestic cats infection is usually asymptomatic. But clinical disease, mainly encephalitis, has been seen in exotic cat species kept in zoological collections, and distemper (or a similar) virus recently caused an epizootic in wild lions in the Serengeti National Park. In addition, there are several reports of CDV as a cause of encephalitis in captive primates.

The so-called 'distemper' viruses of seals and various cetaceans are not canine distemper but related morbilliviruses.

11 INFECTIOUS TRACHEOBRONCHITIS (KENNEL COUGH)

AETIOLOGY

- A number of agents are involved in canine infectious tracheobronchitis – the 'kennel cough' syndrome.
- *Bordetella bronchiseptica* appears to be the major cause.
- A number of viruses may also be involved as primary aetiological agents.
- Combined infections are common.
- Canine distemper virus may also cause predominantly respiratory signs (see preceding chapter) and thus should always be considered as a possible cause of kennel cough, particularly in young, unvaccinated dogs.
- The relative incidence of each of the primary aetiological agents is unknown.
- Other bacteria and mycoplasmas may also be involved in the syndrome, probably mainly as secondary invaders.

Bordetella bronchiseptica

Originally *Bordetella bronchiseptica* was thought to be the cause of canine distemper. Then, when a viral cause of distemper was found, it was thought to be only a secondary pathogen. Now in recent years it has been shown conclusively that it can cause respiratory disease in its own right.

The bacterium appears to attach by means of its fimbriae specifically to the cilia of the trachea and bronchi, and in *in vitro* studies it has been shown that damage to the ciliary cells and ciliostasis occurs. In contrast to other bacteria such as streptococci, *Pasteurella multocida* and staphylococci which are eliminated within 24 hours of experimental infection, *B. bronchiseptica* multiplies rapidly, and after a few days reaches a plateau. As the number of organisms reaches peak levels, clinical signs start to appear. After 2–3 weeks the number of organisms starts to diminish and clinical signs resolve. However some bacteria still persist in the trachea and bronchial tree for several months after infection.

B. bronchiseptica stimulates an acute inflammatory reaction, with muco-purulent discharges present in the trachea and bronchial tree; in some cases there may be lung involvement, though this is uncommon.

Immunity to *B. bronchiseptica* is slow to develop, and the organism is only fully cleared from the respiratory tract by 12–14 weeks after infection. Immunity lasts at least six months, but dogs become susceptible to challenge again by 14 months after infection.

Canine parainfluenza virus (CPIV)

This virus is considered an important cause of kennel cough in the USA and is commonly isolated from outbreaks of the disease. It has also been identified in cases of the disease in Britain, although there is some evidence that it is not as important a cause as *B. bronchiseptica*. Experimentally, the disease is only very mild or subclinical, but in the field, CPIV infection may predispose to combined infections with other viral and/or bacterial agents leading to more typical signs of kennel cough.

The virus replicates mainly in the epithelial cells of the nasal mucosa, pharynx, trachea, large bronchi, and regional lymph nodes, and generalised infection does not occur, except in immunocompromised animals. There may be histopathological lesions in the lung, but these are not important clinically, except where secondary bacterial infection occurs.

Canine adenovirus

There are two distinct canine adenoviruses, canine adenovirus type 1 (CAV-1), which is mainly associated with infectious canine hepatitis (see Chapter 9); and canine adenovirus type 2 (CAV-2), which only seems to be associated with respiratory disease. Both types have been isolated from naturally occurring cases of respiratory disease, and experimentally both can induce mild respiratory disease if given by aerosol. However, CAV-2 is more commonly associated with respiratory disease than CAV-1.

Both viruses induce similar respiratory lesions with a necrotising bronchitis and bronchiolitis and focal necrosis of the turbinates and tonsillar epithelium.

Although lesions are restricted to the respiratory tract, virus can be isolated from both respiratory tract and intestinal epithelium. The normal shedding time for CAV-2 is 8–9 days post infection: although virus can persist in the tissues of clinically recovered dogs for several weeks after infection, unlike in ICH this is probably not epidemiologically important.

Canine herpesvirus (CHV)

This virus can cause a severe generalised disease in neonatal puppies up to 2 weeks of age (see Chapter 14). Thereafter, infection appears to be confined to the respiratory tract, with only very mild signs of upper respiratory disease seen in experimentally infected 3- to 12-week-old pups. Pathological changes are also very mild, but focal epithelial necrosis from nasal and turbinate mucosa through to bronchiolar epithelium may be seen.

CHV has been isolated from dogs with naturally occurring respiratory disease on several occasions, but it is considered a rather uncommon cause of the kennel cough syndrome compared with other viruses such as CPIV and CAV-2. CHV does not seem to spread as easily between dogs as these other viruses, and even in an infected colony not all dogs necessarily become infected: most infections in adult dogs appear to be subclinical. Like other alpha-herpesviruses (e.g. feline herpesvirus, herpes simplex virus), CHV undergoes latent infection in recovered dogs and is sporadically re-excreted.

Canine reovirus

There is serological evidence of all three mammalian serotypes of reovirus infection in the dog population, but little evidence of associated disease. Reoviruses have been isolated from dogs with and without respiratory disease, but Koch's postulates have not been fulfilled. It is unlikely therefore that it is a significant cause of the kennel cough syndrome. However, as it seems to persist in the lymphatic tissues of infected dogs, and it is often found in dual infections with other pathogens, it has been suggested that it may have an immunosuppressive effect that may exacerbate other viral pathogens.

Other possible pathogens

There is some evidence of occasional infections of dogs with influenza viruses, and accompanying signs of respiratory disease. However, there is no good evidence that dogs can infect humans or serve as reservoir hosts for the virus.

Mycoplasmas are commonly found in both diseased and healthy dogs: their main importance is probably as secondary invaders once the respiratory mucosa has been damaged by other, primary agents. However, there is some experimental evidence that *M. cynos* could induce lesions in 1-week-old pups.

CLINICAL SIGNS

- Kennel cough is a highly contagious disease of dogs, and tends to occur where large numbers of dogs are grouped together, for example in boarding kennels and stray-dog homes.
- The incubation period is generally 3–10 days after exposure.
- The syndrome is characterised by the acute onset of an intermittent dry cough, often precipitated by excitement or exercise. Paroxysmal coughing may occur in more severe cases, and in some cases coughing may be followed by gagging or retching. Coughing may be precipitated by pinching the trachea. Dogs generally stay bright and well and continue to eat.
- Some cases show serous or mucopurulent nasal discharge, and some may develop systemic signs such as pyrexia or anorexia.

- Signs usually resolve within 1–3 weeks and recovery is generally uneventful.
- Occasional cases may develop bronchopneumonia. More severe signs are generally seen where there is an uncertain vaccination history, and it is more likely that viruses such as CDV or CAV are involved.

DIAGNOSIS

- Initial diagnosis may often be made from the clinical history. Usually there is a history of recent exposure (e.g. boarding kennels, or rescue kennels), and cases often occur in the summer months when boarding kennel populations are at their peak.
- Vaccination history is useful for helping rule out specific infections, particularly distemper, but it should be remembered that kennel cough is usually multifactorial.
- If the condition does not appear to be infectious, then less common causes of coughing should be considered (e.g. congestive heart failure, allergies, parasites, foreign bodies, etc.).
- Specific viral or bacterial diagnosis is probably not necessary, but can be attempted if required from nasal, pharyngeal or tracheal swabs taken into appropriate transport medium and sent to a specialist laboratory for culture.

Paired serum samples demonstrating rising antibody titres may be used to diagnose *B. bronchiseptica* infection and some of the virus infections. However, vaccinated dogs will already have titres, which can make interpretation difficult. In practice it is difficult to obtain the first serum sample soon enough, unless a sample is available from a susceptible in-contact dog.

Post-mortem examination

Dogs with kennel cough rarely die, but if they do, then specific diagnosis may be achieved in some cases at post-mortem examination.

CDV → characteristic histopathological changes and eosinophilic intracytoplasmic inclusion bodies in lymphoid and epithelial tissues;

CAV → basophilic intranuclear inclusion bodies in respiratory epithelium;

CHV → eosinophilic intranuclear inclusion bodies in respiratory epithelium.

In *B. bronchiseptica* infection many organisms may be seen overlying the ciliated tracheobronchial epithelium.

However, in the absence of specific findings, histopathological diagnosis may be difficult.

In some laboratories, immunofluorescence for particular viral antigens may be undertaken.

TREATMENT

- No antivirals available at present
- If clinical signs mild, specific therapy may not be indicated as disease is usually self-limiting.
- Avoid factors which may precipitate coughing, e.g. exercise and excitement.
- Cough suppressants, e.g. codeine, may be indicated for uncomplicated cases; not where bacterial pneumonia is suspected.
- In general, antibiotics should be given as *B. bronchiseptica* is likely to be involved, and also to control secondary bacterial and mycoplasmal infection. Oxytetracycline or doxycycline are the drugs of choice where *B. bronchiseptica* infection is suspected, but other antibiotics such as trimethoprim–sulphamethoxazole may also be of use. *B. bronchiseptica* tends not to be sensitive to penicillins and cephalosporins.
- In severe cases, aerosol administration of antibiotic may be indicated: particularly in *B. bronchiseptica* infection, oral or parenteral treatment may not give adequate concentrations of antibiotic in the tracheobronchial tree.

PREVENTION AND CONTROL

Vaccination

- No vaccine at present incorporates all known respiratory pathogens, although vaccines are available against the principal pathogens.
- CDV vaccination should be given routinely (for details see preceding chapter).
- CAV vaccination:

  ○ Either CAV-1 or CAV-2 vaccine protect against CAV-1- or CAV-2-induced-respiratory disease (and ICH).
  ○ CAV-2 has now virtually replaced CAV-1 in modified live canine adenovirus vaccines as it does not induce 'blue eye', possible viral persistence with lesions in the kidney, and viral excretion in the urine.
  ○ Inactivated vaccines for CAV infection are also available.
  ○ Maternally derived antibody may interfere with successful vaccination. Thus, although vaccination may be carried out from 6 to 8 weeks of age, a second dose should always be given at 12 weeks of age. Experimental intranasal vaccines have been developed which would overcome MDA, but are not commercially available and in any case are not generally necessary.
  ○ Although immunity following live virus vaccination probably lasts several years, 1- to 2-yearly boosters are generally recommended; annual boosters are required for inactivated vaccines.

- *B. bronchiseptica* vaccination:

  ○ The vaccine currently available against *B. bronchiseptica* is an avirulent strain, given intranasally.

○ It induces a good local IgA immune response and is reasonably effective.

○ The vaccine colonises the respiratory mucosa for several weeks post vaccination, but at a much lower level than the virulent organism.

○ Probably because of the low level of shedding of the avirulent strain, it does not seem to be readily transmitted to in-contact dogs and does not pose any problems.

○ There are few side effects after administration although some dogs may experience transient coughing a few days later.

○ Puppies over 2 weeks of age may be vaccinated since there is no interference with the vaccine by maternally derived antibody.

○ Complete immunity takes 5 days or more to develop after inoculation, and thus dogs should not be exposed before this time: some partial immunity may be present earlier than this.

○ Booster vaccination every 6–10 months is recommended, depending on potential exposure.

○ Dogs being given antibiotics should not be vaccinated.

○ Originally, systemic vaccination against B. bronchiseptica was not found to be consistently satisfactory, with adverse reactions at the injection site being common. However, subunit vaccines are now being developed.

● CPIV vaccination:

○ Modified live vaccines available in UK; intranasal vaccine also available in other countries such as the USA.

○ Vaccines protect against disease, but, although they reduce virus shedding after challenge, they do not eliminate it.

○ Two vaccines given 3–4 weeks apart, with second dose at 12 weeks of age or over.

○ Annual boosters recommended.

Other measures

● Since most of the causative agents are highly contagious, good hygiene and management procedures should also be followed to control the disease.

● The agents are shed in high titre mainly in respiratory secretions of infected dogs, but CAV and CHV are also shed in faeces.

● Spread is via aerosol, by macrodroplets from coughing and sneezing, and by infected secretions on personnel, and feeding and cleaning utensils.

● Thus infected dogs should be isolated and strict hygiene precautions taken to prevent cross-infection.

● Common disinfectants such as hypochlorite and quaternary ammonium compounds are effective.

● Kennel ventilation is very important to reduce the concentration of infectious agents in the atmosphere; 15–20 air changes per hour are recommended.

12 RABIES

Rabies is a neurotropic disease of virtually all mammals which has been recognised since antiquity. It exists world-wide, except where it has been eradicated by quarantine and other measures.

AETIOLOGY

- Caused by a rhabdovirus (Greek *rhabdos* = rod), a bullet-shaped RNA virus with a helical ribonucleocapsid enclosed in a lipid envelope with surface projections.
- Rabies virus belongs to the genus *Lyssavirus* (Greek *lyssa* = madness) in the family Rhabdoviridae.
- For many years, rabies virus was thought to be unique. Conventional serological tests do not readily distinguish strains, and antigenic variation is not important with respect to immunity.
- Monoclonal antibodies can distinguish strains, however, with respect to their species of origin and geographic location.
- There are also several distinct rabies-related viruses which have been isolated in Africa.
- There may be differences in pathogenicity between strains, depending, for example, on their species of origin or on their passage history in the laboratory. Different animal species also vary in their susceptibility to rabies.
- The virus is sensitive to lipid solvents and emulsifying agents, and thus is quickly inactivated by a number of disinfectants including formalin, soap and quaternary ammonium compounds. It is easily inactivated by heat and sunlight, but is stable at low temperatures. Under normal environmental conditions, therefore, it does not remain infective for long outside the host.

TRANSMISSION

- Rabies virus is excreted in the saliva of infected animals and is almost always transmitted by biting; occasionally it may be transmitted by contamination of mucosa or a superficial wound.

- Airborne transmission recorded in the USA in man, coyotes and foxes (but not in dogs and cats) following exposure to infected bats in caves.
- Oral infection achieved experimentally in a number of species including foxes, skunks and cats, and infection of dogs from eating rabid fox carcasses also reported.

PATHOGENESIS

The susceptibility of animals to rabies virus varies a great deal and depends on factors such as:

the animal species
its genetic make-up
the age of the animal
the virus strain (biotype)
the virus dose
the route of exposure.

For example, a deep, heavily contaminated wound in the head region in a young animal is more likely to lead to disease, with a shorter incubation period, than in an older animal with a superficial wound on the extremities.

The incubation period
This is very variable and depends on factors such as those outlined above. Under experimental conditions in dogs the range is 9–125 days (mean 24 days) and in cats 9–51 days (median 18 days).

Under natural conditions the incubation period is generally 1–2 months though in some instances it may be much longer, up to 6 months. In dogs, cases have occasionally been recorded beyond this time.

The pathogenesis of infection is shown in Figure 12.1.

CLINICAL SIGNS

The clinical course is classically described as three, often overlapping phases:

(1) the prodromal period;
(2) the excitative or 'furious' stage;
(3) the paralytic or 'dumb' phase.

However, not all animals progress through all these stages and the presentation can be quite variable.

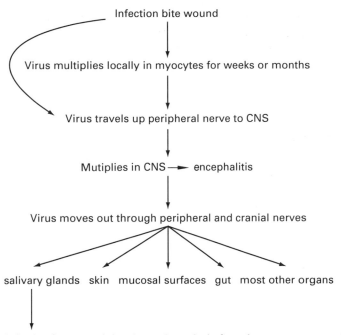

Infection bite wound

Virus multiplies locally in myocytes for weeks or months

Virus travels up peripheral nerve to CNS

Mutiplies in CNS ➝ encephalitis

Virus moves out through peripheral and cranial nerves

salivary glands   skin   mucosal surfaces   gut   most other organs

Saliva infective for several days/up to 2 weeks before signs appear ➝ death

Figure 12.1 The pathogenesis of rabies

Prodromal period

- This may last for 2–3 days in dogs, but only a day or two in cats, and is characterised by a marked change in behaviour.
- Animals may appear anxious, uneasy and irritable, and may have increased sensitivity to noise and light.
- Sullen animals may become more alert, restless and friendly, whereas more amicable ones may become aggressive and attack without provocation, or become depressed and withdrawn, hiding in dark places.
- Aggression is more commonly seen in cats than in dogs.
- During this initial period there may be slight pyrexia and some dilatation of the pupils with impaired corneal reflex.
- Animals may self-mutilate at the site of the bite.

Excitative stage

- Gradually the excitement phase predominates.
- Animals become increasingly nervous, irritable and vicious, and are most likely to bite and attack. Disorientation: 'far-off look in the eyes'.
- Muscle tremors, flaccidity or incoordination usually develop.

- As in humans, spasm and eventual paralysis of the muscles of deglutition lead to difficulty in swallowing, and drooling and frothing of saliva.
- Dogs may also show pica, i.e. eating unusual objects such as wood, and they may develop a characteristic high-toned bark as laryngeal paralysis ensues.
- The excitement phase may last up to a week, but sometimes animals progress directly from the prodromal phase to the paralytic stage.

Paralytic phase

- Muscular incoordination and convulsions gradually lead to generalised paralysis, coma and death.

Atypical rabies/carrier state

Although in classical rabies animals progress straight through the clinical signs to death, there are rare reports of recovery. A carrier state has been reported in dogs in Ethiopia, and there is some evidence for this in cats also.

PATHOLOGY

Gross

Minimal pathological findings. The carcass may be emaciated; there may be evidence of self-trauma; and in dogs particularly there may be foreign bodies in the alimentary tract because of pica.

Histopathology

- Diffuse encephalitis with mononuclear cell perivascular cuffing and focal gliosis, i.e. an inflammatory response typical of any non-suppurative infection of the brain. Spongiform lesions in the brains of rabid animals have also been reported.
- Neuronal degeneration in rabies is relatively severe compared with some other viral infections of the CNS, particularly in carnivores.
- *Negri bodies*. Neurones may contain the pathognomonic intracytoplasmic inclusions: 'Negri bodies'. These may occur in several areas of the brain but are most prominent in the hippocampus. In cats some confusion may arise as similar inclusions may be seen in some nerve cells in normal cats. Negri bodies were used extensively in diagnosis of rabies, but this has now been superseded in most countries by more reliable and rapid techniques.
- Other changes are minimal but may include ganglioneuritis in the para-vertebral ganglia and possible degenerative changes in the salivary gland.

DIAGNOSIS

- Furious form easiest to diagnose: should be distinguished from pseudorabies (Aujeszky's disease).
- Incoordinate, paralytic or moribund animal most difficult to diagnose.

Differential diagnosis

Differential diagnosis includes:

- toxoplasmosis;
- CNS infection;
- feline infectious peritonitis;
- canine distemper;
- neoplasia;
- trauma;
- hepatic encephalopathy;
- thiamine deficiency (cats);
- oral and pharyngeal foreign bodies;
- poisoning with, for example, lead, organochloride compounds, benzoic acid (cats), strychnine;
- spongiform encephalopathy (cats);
- general weakness seen in moribund animals from various generalised infections.

Action to be taken in the UK in a case of suspected rabies

- Detain animal on premises.
- Notify local divisional veterinary officer of the Ministry of Agriculture.
- Veterinary surgeon and handlers should carry out personal disinfection with soap or detergent (not both) and water, and change contaminated clothing.
- If bitten or scratched, flush wound immediately with soap or detergent (not both) and water, then water alone, then apply 40–70% alcohol, tincture or aqueous solutions of iodine, or 0.1% quaternary ammonium compound (e.g. cetrimide BP).
- No further animals should enter the waiting room until case diagnosed negative or satisfactory cleansing and disinfection of premises has taken place under supervision of Ministry veterinary officer.
- Names and addresses of any contacts (e.g. those in waiting room) should be recorded. The veterinary officer will inform the medical officer for environmental health for any further action.
- If the animal dies or is killed, its head and neck should be removed by a Ministry veterinary officer and transported fresh and intact in a sealed container held at a low temperature, but not frozen, to an appropriate diagnostic laboratory (in the UK, the Central Veterinary Laboratory, Weybridge).

Laboratory diagnosis

- A combination of several diagnostic techniques is generally used to diagnose rabies.
- Fluorescent antibody on brain smears to demonstrate viral antigen. Results in 2–3 hours, high degree of accuracy.
- Histological examination of brain material, usually from hippocampus, for specific Negri inclusion bodies. Results in 2 days, but not very accurate and in most countries now superseded by other tests.
- Examination of formalin-fixed brain tissue by immunochemical techniques or, if trypsin treated, by immunofluorescence.
- Mouse inoculation: mice inoculated intracerebrally with suspension of brain tissue, and brains examined by immunofluorescence at intervals up to 28 days post inoculation.
- Cell cultures: in recent years, some cell lines have been found to be equally if not more sensitive than mouse inoculation for diagnosis and have now superseded it in many laboratories.
- Panels of monoclonal antibodies may be used in immunofluorescence tests on brain smears or infected cell cultures to determine the origin of the rabies virus (i.e. vaccine or field, rabies or rabies-related virus, or which species it comes from, e.g. skunk or fox).
- Detection of rabies virus by polymerase chain reaction (PCR) recently described.

EPIDEMIOLOGY

Although virtually every mammal is susceptible to rabies, the natural disease occurs predominantly in carnivores. In different geographic areas, usually only one or two species predominate as vectors.

- In Europe, the red fox is the most important reservoir host and vector. The fox population undergoes both annual and seasonal variations in cycles of infection. When the incidence of rabies increases in foxes, it also increases in domestic species such as cattle, sheep, cats and dogs. Human exposure occurs through contact with infected domestic animals.

  Oral vaccination of foxes using baits which contain live attenuated rabies vaccines or a recombinant vaccinia–rabies virus is now being undertaken and looks very promising. Where fox rabies or foxes are eliminated, the disease disappears from all other species (except bats). Bat rabies in Europe exists largely as an independent cycle and only occasionally does spill-over to terrestrial mammals occur.

- In the USA and Canada, rabies is enzootic in several species such as skunks, foxes and raccoons, from which it may pass to domestic animals and then man. Bat rabies also occurs but, as in Europe, only occasionally leads to infection in other species.

- In South America, rabies is enzootic in both wildlife (i.e. sylvatic rabies) and dogs (urban rabies). Vampire bats are the most frequent source of infection to cattle, and dogs are the major vector for humans. Control of the disease in the dog population by vaccination leads to a marked drop in human exposure.
- In Eastern Europe, Africa and Asia, both wildlife and urban rabies also co-exist. A number of wildlife species including wolves, jackals and mongooses act as reservoir hosts, filling the same ecological niche that foxes do in other countries.

PREVENTION AND CONTROL

There are several aspects to be considered here.

Preventative vaccination for humans

Originally, inactivated vaccines were prepared from nervous systems of animals but these led to adverse reactions. In developed countries they have now been superseded by inactivated vaccines derived from cell cultures. Recombinant vaccines (e.g. canarypox) are also being developed. Veterinarians and others exposed to an increased risk should be protected by vaccination.

Post-exposure treatment for humans

Post-exposure treatment requires several vaccinations plus an injection of specific immunoglobulin at the same time as the first vaccine if the exposure was severe.

Preventative vaccination for domestic animals

Originally live attenuated vaccines were used, but because of safety considerations they have now been largely superseded by inactivated vaccines. Primary vaccination is not generally recommended before 3 months of age, and should be followed by a booster 1 year later. Thereafter annual or triennial boosters should be given. One month should be allowed for the development of immunity.

It should be remembered that fully vaccinated animals may in some cases still develop rabies.

Recombinant (vaccinia and other poxvirus) vaccines have also recently been shown to be safe and efficacious in several species.

Post-exposure treatment for animals

In animals generally only preventive vaccination is carried out. However, in some countries post-exposure treatment may be allowed but only if the animal has previously been vaccinated.

SECTION 2

Preventative vaccination for reservoir hosts

Oral vaccination of foxes using bait containing live attenuated rabies vaccines or a recombinant vaccinia–rabies virus is now being undertaken. Both types of vaccine appear to work well and many areas of Europe are now free of rabies. The recombinant vaccine may have advantages of safety and stability over the attenuated vaccine. It has also been shown to be safe and efficacious for the oral immunisation of the main vectors in North America.

Other control measures

In some countries free of rabies, the disease is excluded by quarantine. For example, in the UK, animals such as dogs and cats have to undergo a 6-month quarantine period on arrival, in kennels which are under veterinary supervision and are approved and inspected by Ministry of Agriculture veterinary officers. All animals entering quarantine are required to be vaccinated, with an approved vaccine. Recently, EU regulations now allow commercially traded animals, which come from a registered holding, to move freely between member states, including the UK. However, certain conditions apply regarding the identification of animals, and there must be evidence of successful vaccination having been carried out.

In countries where rabies is enzootic, control measures should be aimed at reducing the incidence of disease in cats and dogs and in wildlife, i.e.:

- stray dogs and cats should be eliminated;
- dogs and cats should be licensed;
- the movement of animals should be restricted;
- vaccination should be carried out, preferably with inactivated vaccines.

In wildlife, although measures such as destroying foxes have been tried, they are only temporarily effective because the fox population rapidly recovers and rabies then recurs. Undoubtedly the most successful means of rabies control in wildlife is by vaccination using oral baits.

13 CANINE PAPILLOMAVIRUS INFECTION

CLINICAL SIGNS

Canine papillomavirus infection is fairly common in puppies, in which it causes oral papillomas. Found world-wide.

- Initially smooth, pale, or pink, papules, which later develop into larger, irregular, cauliflower-like lesions.
- Usually limited to buccal mucosa and tongue, and occasionally conjunctivae.
- Benign and self limiting (usually recover in 1–5 months).
- Sometimes interferes with eating, or associated with halitosis or mild oral haemorrhage.
- Rarely affects the oesophagus or skin around nose and mouth.

Cutaneous papillomas and warts in older dogs may also be caused by a papilloma virus, but if so the virus appears to be different, and not so readily transmissible as that associated with oral papillomas in puppies.

DIAGNOSIS

Diagnosis is generally made from the clinical signs, but can be confirmed by histopathology, especially immunocytochemistry. Like most papillomaviruses, canine papillomavirus cannot be grown in cell culture.

TREATMENT

Treatment is usually unnecessary, but if the tumours are causing discomfort or obstruction, or persist, surgical removal may be indicated. Care must be taken not to spread lesions by inoculation of infective material into fresh sites during surgery. The value of autogenous vaccines in affected animals is debatable, although some experimental vaccines have provoked good protective immunity.

CONTROL

Commercial or specially produced autogenous vaccines are available in some areas, but are only recommended for use during outbreaks in large kennels.

14   CANINE HERPESVIRUS INFECTION

AETIOLOGY

Canine herpesvirus (CHV) is an occasional cause of fading puppy syndrome, upper respiratory tract disease (kennel cough) (see Chapter 11) and abortion/ stillbirths in dogs. The main route of transmission appears to be oronasal from infected puppies or from nasal or vaginal excretions of adults. The virus spreads rapidly through kennels but usually only causes disease in very young puppies.

Infection of adults or puppies over 3 weeks old results in replication in the respiratory tract without clinical disease. The virus can undergo latent infection and reactivation, and further shedding can be induced by immunosuppression or stress.

In very young puppies, the virus generalises by viraemia, and replicates in many organs including the CNS.

Age resistance appears to be mainly a matter of body temperature: the virus grows best at temperatures just below that of normal dogs, so puppies less than 3 weeks old, which generally cannot yet regulate their own temperature, are most at risk of generalised disease.

CLINICAL SIGNS

- In very young puppies include:

  - anorexia;
  - soft stools progressing to diarrhoea;
  - painful abdomen: the puppies cry continually with paddling limb movements until they die;
  - sometimes dyspnoea;
  - vomiting or salivation.

- Most puppies less than 2–3 weeks old die within 1 or 2 days of onset of clinical signs.
- Sudden death in very young puppies may be due to CHV infection.
- 'Fading puppy syndrome'.

- Puppies over 2 weeks old seldom become severely ill, but may develop respiratory signs (see page 90).
- Occassionally vesicular lesions on male and female genitalia in adults.
- Abortion or stillborn puppies from bitches infected during pregnancy.
- Most infection of adults is subclinical.

DIAGNOSIS

Diagnosis of CHV infection of puppies is usually made at necropsy.

- Characteristic petechial haemorrhage and focal necrosis produce speckled kidneys.
- Inclusion bodies seen by histological examination and virus isolation are necessary for confirmation.

In adults, diagnosis is difficult as virus is quite labile and excreted only occasionally and in small amounts, while antibody levels are often very low or undetectable.

TREATMENT AND CONTROL

- Keep small puppies in warm environment to raise body temperature to above 38.5°C.
- No vaccine available.
- Subsequent litters rarely affected due to protection afforded by maternal antibody.

15 LEPTOSPIROSIS

AETIOLOGY

Dogs can be infected with several serovars of *Leptospira interrogans*, but those most often found are *icterohaemorrhagiae*, *canicola* and *grippotyphosa*. The sources of infection in dogs are usually environmental – particularly slow moving water and contact with rodents, but also bite wounds, infected meat and even placental transfer.

A combination of hygiene and vaccination means that canine leptospirosis is not commonly reported in many areas. Affected dogs are usually unvaccinated with a history of swimming in stagnant or slow-moving water.

PATHOGENESIS AND CLINICAL SIGNS (Figure 15.1)

- Leptospires usually enter through mucous membranes or broken skin. Replicate in blood, renal tubules and liver.
- Disease depends on dose and serovar of leptospire and on age of dog and degree of immunity: pre-existing high antibody titre leads to elimination of organism, moderate antibody to mild or asymptomatic infection.
- Full blown peracute clinical disease is generally seen only in unvaccinated dogs.
- Peracute disease due to massive leptospiraemia: pyrexia, shivering, muscle tenderness, vomiting, dehydration, shock and death.
- Sub-acute infections – fever, anorexia, vomiting and dehydration. May be reluctant to move owing to abdominal pain. Mucous membranes congested, possible petechial haemorrhage. Infection of kidney then leads to progressive loss of renal function – oliguria and anuria.
- Dogs which eliminate infection may return to normal in 2–3 weeks. But widespread damage may lead to chronic renal failure. Hepatic infection may lead to jaundice and chronic hepatitis.
- Most infections, however, are chronic rather than acute or subacute, with rather vaguer clinical signs such as pyrexia, or progressive chronic renal or hepatic failure.
- Infected dogs may excrete leptospires in urine for months or even years.

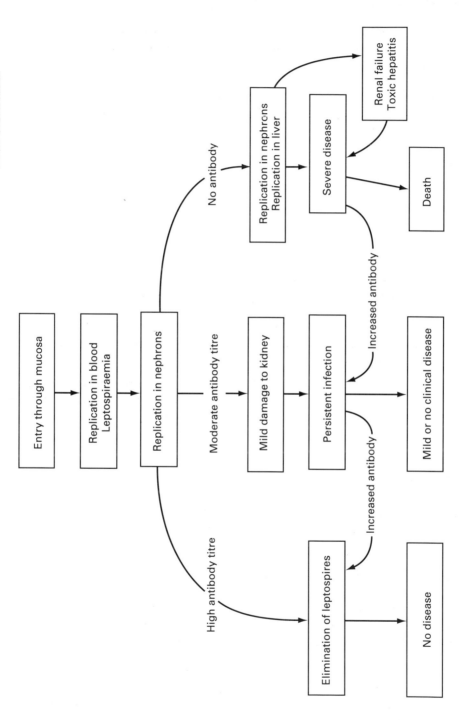

Figure 15.1 The pathogenesis of canine leptospirosis

DIAGNOSIS

Diagnosis is often based on clinical signs and history (environment and lack of vaccine), supported by haematology (leucocytosis, thrombocytopenia) and blood biochemistry (urea and creatinine levels raised, elevated liver enzymes and bilirubin).

Serology is expensive and can be difficult to interpret.

Isolation from urine and blood is difficult as leptospires do not survive long and need special transport media. The organism can also sometimes be seen in urine by dark-ground microscopy.

Leptospires can also be detected by immunofluorescence in liver or kidney sections snap-frozen in liquid nitrogen then sent frozen to the laboratory.

TREATMENT

Antibiotic therapy:

- Penicillin G (25 mg/kg IV or IM twice daily) or ampicillin (10 mg/kg IV, IM or SC twice daily, or 10–20 mg/kg orally three times daily) for 2 weeks to control bacteraemia.
- Dihydrostreptomycin (15 mg/kg, IM or SC twice daily) for 2 weeks to eliminate renal infection. *Only use streptomycin once renal function has returned to normal.*

Supportive therapy, including rehydration and/or blood transfusion can be used if necessary, and possibly diuretics or even peritoneal dialysis in persistently oliguric animals. Appropriate low-protein diets can help in the management of renal failure.

CONTROL

Control is mainly by vaccination with killed *L. interrogans icterohaemorrhagiae* and *canicola* and avoidance of contaminated environments.

PUBLIC HEALTH ASPECTS

The leptospires which infect dogs and cats can also infect and cause severe, sometimes fatal disease (Weil's disease) in man. The zoonotic potential of the infection must always be kept in mind if leptospirosis is suspected in a dog or cat.

However, dogs (and, presumably, cats) are relatively rare sources of human infection nowadays. The most frequent sources of human infection are rat-infested environments – there is a relatively high risk of infection amongst those taking part in water sports – and cattle.

FELINE LEPTOSPIROSIS

Clinical leptospirosis is very rare in cats, although antibody has been demonstrated in about 7% of cats in the UK. Various serovars have been detected, including *icterohaemorrhagiae*, *pomona* and *bratislava*.

Pathogenesis of experimental leptospirosis in cats is similar to that in dogs, yet clinical signs rarely appear except at the histological level.

Cats have been shown to be capable of excreting the organism in urine for up to 3 months following experimental infection.

16 CANINE BRUCELLOSIS

AETIOLOGY

Brucella canis can cause abortion and epididymitis in dogs, fading puppy syndrome, and sometimes systemic disease, osteomyelitis, discospondylitis or even meningoencephalitis. *B. canis* is especially common in Central and South America and the southern USA, but is not normally found in the UK.

Canine brucellosis is mainly spread through contact with vaginal discharges during and after abortion, although urine can also contain the organism. Males can transmit *B. canis* in semen for several months.

CLINICAL SIGNS

- Abortion of partially autolysed fetuses at 45–55 days of gestation.
- Early embryonic death may also occur but is usually missed and the bitch will be presented as having failed to conceive.
- In males there may be scrotal swelling due to epididymitis and loss of fertility.
- Constant licking may lead to moist dermatitis on scrotum.
- May also see lethargy, generalised lymphadenitis and loss of libido.
- Rarely, infection has also been associated with osteomyelitis, discospondylitis or recurrent uveitis.

DIAGNOSIS

Serological tests are rapid and relatively cheap, but most have a high rate (up to 50%) of false positives.

Blood culture is both sensitive and specific and is the laboratory test of choice, although time consuming.

TREATMENT

Treatment is expensive and often unsuccessful, especially if not instigated early in infection.

Suggested protocols

- tetracycline (25 mg/kg three times daily orally) and streptomycin (10 mg/kg twice daily by intramuscular injection) combined for 1 week, followed by continuation of tetracycline for a further 3 weeks; or
- doxycycline (12.5 mg/kg twice daily orally) for 2 weeks with gentamicin (2 mg/kg subcutaneous or intramuscular injection twice daily) for 1 week.

The whole treatment may need repeating, particularly for treatment of localised infections (e.g. in the eye).

CONTROL

Control is based on annual testing of all dogs in a colony and testing of all dogs twice (4–6 weeks apart) before they are allowed into a colony.

There is no vaccine available.

Section 3
MISCELLANEOUS VIRAL INFECTIONS

17 AUJESZKY'S DISEASE/ PSEUDORABIES

AETIOLOGY

Aujeszky's disease (also known as pseudorabies and mad itch) is caused by a herpesvirus, *Herpesvirus suis*. Although pigs are the reservoir host, other animals, for example cattle, sheep, dogs, cats and rats, can also be infected. These species are 'dead end' hosts, however, and do not generally transmit the disease themselves, although cats and dogs may shed virus in their oral and nasal secretions.

Infection in dogs and cats is usually associated with contact with infected pigs or eating uncooked, infected pig meat. Note that in some areas of the world this may include wild pig meat, e.g. wild boars.

CLINICAL SIGNS

- Almost always fatal, and often rapidly so.
- First clinical signs seen in cats and dogs are usually behavioural changes: restlessness, anorexia and hypersalivation.
- Some dogs appear overexcited, continually barking.
- Often no clinical signs seen in cats as they run off to hide early in disease development.
- Intense pruritus, commonly localised around the face or mouth is often described as a characteristic sign of Aujeszky's disease in dogs.
- May become frenzied in an attempt to alleviate the intolerable itching, and gross self-mutilation can often result. It is in this form that the disease may be mistaken for rabies, but unlike rabid animals, cats and dogs with Aujeszky's disease are rarely aggressive.
- But many infected animals are not pruritic.
- Terminal signs usually within 48 hours of the onset of clinical signs, include paralysis and coma.
- Some cats and dogs may die suddenly without showing any prior clinical signs.

DIAGNOSIS

Diagnosis is usually made at necropsy, as progression of disease is so fast that antibody has not developed by time of death.

Virus can sometimes be isolated from tonsil, spleen or brain. More sensitive, however, is demonstration of virus antigen in frozen sections of tonsil or brain.

SECTION 3

18 HANTAVIRUS INFECTION

Hantaviruses are enzootic world-wide in wild and laboratory rodent populations, and are often zoonotic. Strains of *Hantavirus* differ in their virulence in man. The hantavirus pulmonary syndrome in North America and haemorrhagic fever with renal syndrome in Asia both cause high mortality. However, most European strains usually induce only subclinical or mild disease.

Hantavirus antibody in cats was first detected in laboratory-housed cats and dogs in Belgium, and virus has been isolated from a cat in China. Recent surveys in Britain and Austria found antibody reactive to *Hantavirus* in up to 10% of cats from a variety of disease and environmental backgrounds, but a similar survey in The Netherlands did not detect any antibody.

The clinical significance of *Hantavirus* infection in cats is not known, and there is little evidence to suggest that cats are a source of human infection in the West; the overall prevalence of antibody in man in the UK is only 0.5% with higher prevalences found in those whose work or recreation exposes them to rodents.

19 FELINE ROTAVIRUS INFECTION

Rotaviruses are a well established cause of acute diarrhoea in many mammalian species, for example humans, cattle, sheep and pigs, but there are few reports of rotavirus infection in cats, and it is probably not a major cause of feline enteric disease.

- Subclinical infection is probably most common.
- Diarrhoea is most likely to be seen in young kittens, but is usually only mild and transient.
- More severe disease may occur in the presence of other pathogens or predisposing factors, or in large, intensively housed colonies where high levels of virus may accumulate in the environment.
- Diagnosis is usually by electron microscopy (EM) of faeces, although polyacrylamide gel electrophoresis has been described and is very useful for diagnosing rotavirus infections in other species.
- The commercially available ELISA kits for detecting rotavirus in human and bovine faeces may not detect feline strains of rotavirus.

Treatment, if necessary, is symptomatic.

Although rotaviruses can cross species, cats are an unlikely source of human rotavirus infection.

20   FELINE REOVIRUS INFECTION

Reoviruses are found in many mammalian and avian species and can be divided into three serotypes regardless of species of origin. The clinical importance of infection in cats is unknown, although serological surveys show that infection is widespread.

- Reoviruses have been isolated from the faeces and oropharyngeal secretions of cats showing a variety of clinical signs and also from healthy cats.
- Experimentally:

  ○ Inoculation of new-born kittens with reovirus type 1 caused death in 2 days. Necropsy revealed signs of respiratory infection.
  ○ Inoculation of kittens with reovirus type 2 caused mild diarrhoea.
  ○ Inoculation of kittens with reovirus type 3 induced mild conjunctivitis and respiratory signs.

- Diagnosis is by detection of virus from faeces or oropharyngeal swabs by EM or isolation using special cell culture techniques.
- Control measures are probably not indicated because infection is thought to be subclinical or, at most, mild.

SECTION 3

21   FELINE ASTROVIRUS INFECTION

Astroviruses are small RNA viruses with a characteristic five- or six-pointed star-shaped morphology.

Little has been published on the epidemiology or clinical significance of feline astrovirus infection. One report suggests that less than 10% cats in the UK have antibody.

- Green and watery diarrhoea lasting 4–14 days, sometimes accompanied by vomiting, pyrexia and depression.
- Diagnosis is by electron microscopy of faeces.
- Treatment is symptomatic.

22 FELINE TOROVIRUS INFECTION

Toroviruses are a group of viruses similar to the coronaviruses, but with a characteristic rod or doughnut-shaped core. They include Berne virus, isolated from a horse, Breda virus isolated from cattle, and several torovirus-like isolates from humans.

Recently, torovirus-like particles and antibody reacting with Breda virus types 1 and 2 have also been detected in cats.

Although not reproduced experimentally, there is some evidence to link this virus in cats to a clinical syndrome involving persistent diarrhoea and protrusion of the nictitating membrane.

23 FELINE SYNCYTIUM-FORMING VIRUS INFECTION

Feline syncytium-forming virus (FeSFV) is a member of the foamy virus group (the Spumavirinae) in the family Retroviridae. FeSFV infection is extremely common in cats. The virus infects many cell types in many organs of the body, and is excreted in saliva.

Other spumaviruses have been isolated from many species but, unlike the oncoviruses and lentiviruses, they do not appear to be pathogenic, although an involvement of FeSFV in feline polyarthritis has been suggested. Their main importance at present lies not in clinical medicine but as potential contaminants of cell cultures used in research and for vaccine production.

24 FELINE PARAPOXVIRUS INFECTION

Several anecdotal accounts and one well documented report exist of feline parapoxvirus (orf) infection. The condition appears to be less common than feline cowpox. In the best recorded case, the infected cat had multiple, crusty and scabbed skin lesions which healed after several weeks, and the cat had been in contact with goats. Diagnosis depends on electron microscopy of scabs as parapoxviruses are difficult to grow in cell culture.

25 FELINE HERPESVIRUS TYPE 2 INFECTION

FHV-2 is a cell-associated feline herpesvirus, serologically distinct from feline herpesvirus 1. It was apparently isolated from a cat with feline urological syndrome (FUS), and it was suggested that it might be implicated in the aetiology of the syndrome. Other workers, however, have been unable to transmit FUS, and have failed to isolate a similar agent. Serum antibody to the original isolate has apparently been detected in 30% of cats in the USA, but not in cat sera in the UK. Antigenic and molecular studies on FHV-2 have shown it to be identical to bovid herpesvirus 4 (BHV-4). BHV-4 has been isolated from cattle with respiratory and reproductive disease, and the European type strain of BHV-4 has been shown not to be infectious for domestic cats. The origin and significance of the American cat isolate remain unknown.

26 FELINE 'STAGGERING DISEASE'

A neurological syndrome of cats characterised by unsteady 'staggering' gait, depression, and progressive hindlimb ataxia and paresis has been described from several European countries, and possibly other parts of the world including North

America and Australia. Post-mortem examination reveals a very characteristic non-suppurative meningoencephalomyelitis mainly in the grey matter of the cortex, brain stem and spinal cord. The histopathology is consistent with a viral infection, and, although the causative virus has not yet been isolated, affected cats have high antibody titre to Borna disease virus (BDV). BDV is the cause of a progressive encephalopathy of horses and sheep in Central Europe, and BDV or a related virus has also been associated with certain psychiatric disorders in man.

27 CANINE ACIDOPHIL CELL HEPATITIS

An apparently uncommon form of acute or chronic transmissible hepatitis in the dog, believed to be caused by a virus. Initial clinical signs are vague, but typical signs of chronic liver failure eventually develop: vomiting, abdominal pain, ascites, neurological signs of hepatic encephalopathy, coma and death. Very little has been published on this disease.

28 CANINE CALICIVIRUS INFECTIONS

Caliciviruses associated with diarrhoea in dogs have been mentioned earlier, but caliciviruses have also been isolated from dogs associated with glossitis and with vaginal vesicles.

29 CANINE RETROVIRUS INFECTIONS

There are several reports of retrovirus-like particles and reverse transcriptase activity in various canine tissues and cell lines, and retrovirus-like sequences have been detected in the dog genome. Only recently, however, has a lentivirus-like retrovirus been isolated in cell culture from a dog. The epidemiology and clinical significance of this virus are not known.

30 OTHER VIRAL INFECTIONS

- *Influenza virus* can infect cats following experimental inoculation, and there is some serological evidence of infection in the field. However, there is no evidence that cat to human transmission might occur, the reverse being more likely during human influenza pandemics. Influenza virus has also been isolated from dogs and may cause mild upper respiratory tract disease. The source of infection is probably also humans.
- *Paramyxovirus* infection of the CNS has been described in cats associated with demyelinating encephalitis and with clinical neurological signs. Antibody to mumps has been reported in dogs, but this may simply be due to serological cross-reaction with canine parainfluenza virus. Canine distemper virus (CDV) can also infect domestic cats both experimentally and in the field but generally causes no clinical signs. In big cats, however, natural CDV infection has been associated with encephalitis (see page 88).
- *Arthropod-borne virus* (particularly alpha- and flavivirus) infection of both cats and dogs has been reported from various parts of the world. Infection is usually asymptomatic but occasionally causes encephalitis, for example louping ill in dogs which is transmitted by ixodid ticks.
- A *herpesvirus* closely related to feline herpesvirus1 (page 3) has been isolated from a dog with diarrhoea, but the significance of this virus in terms of prevalence and pathogenicity is not known.

- Various *human enteroviruses* have been isolated from dogs without being associated with disease, and again humans are thought to be the source of infection.
- *Lymphochoriomeningitis virus* is a virus found in mice and is only rarely transmitted to man. However, there are some old reports showing that dogs can be experimentally infected with LCMV. Furthermore these dogs were able to infect other dogs sharing their kennels. So dogs can be infected and shed infectious virus. Whether this has any epidemiological or zoonotic significance in the field is not known.

Section 4
MISCELLANEOUS BACTERIAL INFECTIONS

31 FELINE ABSCESS AND CELLULITIS

AETIOLOGY

Infection often involves several bacterial species. Anaerobes and facultative anaerobes most frequently isolated include:

Pasteurella multocida
Bacteroides spp
Streptococcus spp
Fusobacterium spp
Actinomyces spp
E. coli
Nocardia asteroides
Rhodococcus equi
Dermatophilus congolensis
Mycoplasma spp
Mycobacterium spp

Fungi are sometimes found, mainly as secondary invaders in chronic abscesses, for example:

Candida spp
Microsporum spp
Trichophyton spp
Trichosporon spp
Hyphomycetes
Sporothrix schenki

Occasionally viruses may also be isolated from abscesses, for example:

cowpox virus
feline herpesvirus-1 (FHV-1)
feline calicivirus (FCV)

Cowpox virus may be part of the cause of cellulitis or a persistent abscess. Both FHV and FCV can cause skin ulceration, but they are usually regarded as contaminants if isolated from an abscess rather than the cause of the lesion. They are probably transmitted in saliva from the oropharynx by the cat licking at its wound.

EPIDEMIOLOGY

Abscesses and cellulitis are probably the most common infections encountered in cats. They are mostly due to bites and scratches from fighting with other cats, or occasionally with rodents. The possibility of foreign bodies, including grass seed-heads and airgun pellets, should also be investigated.

As might be expected, bite abscesses are more common in males, particularly non-castrated males, than in females and are more common in cats which roam rather than those kept in the house.

CLINICAL SIGNS

- Clinical signs vary according to the site and severity of the lesion.
- Bite or scratch wounds are generally found on the head, leg, back or base of tail.
- Usually painful, giving rise to:
  - altered gait
  - guarding of the site
  - altered behaviour including depression, inappetance, and aggression.
- Cats may be pyrexic and have enlarged local lymph nodes.
- Mature abscesses can be palpated but may not be so obvious early in their development.
- Possible sequelae depend on the site of the lesions, the organisms involved and the immune status of the cat. They include:
  - pyothorax
  - osteomyelitis
  - rhinitis
  - otitis
  - meningitis
  - pyaemia with localisation at distant sites
  - bacterial endocarditis (rare).
- If abscesses persist or recur, unusual organisms such as mycobacteria, immunosuppression by feline immunodeficiency virus or feline leukaemia virus infection or a hidden foreign body should be suspected.

DIAGNOSIS

- Largely by clinical signs and careful examination.
- Haematology may help.

TREATMENT

Treatment depends on extent of infection and stage of development of abscess.

Antibiotics

Antibiotics are generally unable to penetrate abscess walls, but may be useful for treating cellulitis and help prevent recurrence after drainage and other complications.

- A single injection of penicillin G (25 mg/kg IM) given within 24 hours of being bitten may help prevent cellulitis and abscess formation.
- Penicillins and their derivatives such as ampicillin and amoxycillin (both at 20 mg/kg orally three times daily) are effective against most abscess-forming bacteria.
- Second- or third-generation cephalosporins (e.g. cefoxitin at 10–20 mg/kg SC three times daily), clindamycin (10 mg/kg orally twice daily) and metronidazole (10 mg/kg orally three times daily) are second choice for their particular activity against anaerobes.

Surgical drainage

- This should be done after, and only after, the abscess has matured. Maturation may be enhanced by warm saline compresses.
- Drained abscesses can be debrided if necessary, cleaned with, for example, dilute hydrogen peroxide or proprietary antiseptic and cleansing solutions, then left open for drainage.

SECTION 4

32 ACTINOMYCOSIS AND NOCARDIOSIS

AETIOLOGY

Both *Actinomyces* spp and *Nocardia* spp are Gram-positive, pleomorphic, branching rods and filaments. The two organisms are difficult to distinguish except by culture.

Actinomyces are part of the normal flora of the oral cavity and respiratory tract of cats and dogs.

Nocardia are common soil saprophytes.

CLINICAL SIGNS

- Persistent pyogranulomatous lesions.
- Most frequently isolated from abscesses, cellulitis and pyothorax.
- *Actinomyces* infection is about 10 times as common as *Nocardia* and is particularly associated with bite wounds, although any wound can become infected simply by licking.
- Pus caused by either organism frequently contains 'sulphur granules'.

TREATMENT

Both can be difficult to treat and, whatever the site of the lesion, drainage and removal of pus is essential for effective antibiotic therapy.

Actinomyces spp are usually susceptible to long-term treatment with penicillins but not metronidazole.

Nocardia spp are often sensitive only to sulphonamides with or without trimethoprim potentiation.

Although antibiotic treatment is usually started before these organisms have been isolated, antibiotic sensitivity tests are recommended to ensure that the optimum antibiotic is used.

33 MYCETOMA

Mycetomas are chronic pyogranulomatous actinomycotic or mycotic infections of the skin and deeper tissues which form firm, often large and multiple masses, possibly with discharging sinuses.

Various oral or soil organisms such as *Actinomyces*, *Nocardia* and *Streptomyces* spp may be involved in actinomycotic mycetomas.

Mycotic mycetomas are rare in cats and dogs but there are reports of cases involving *Torula* spp and *Microsporum canis*.

Therapy includes radical surgical resection and antibiotic (see page 128) or antifungal therapy (ketoconazole at 5–10 mg/kg orally three times daily or griseofulvin at 15–30 mg/kg orally daily) but is often unsuccessful.

34 TUBERCULOSIS

AETIOLOGY

Dogs and cats can be infected with *Mycobacterium tuberculosis*, *M. bovis*, *M. avium* or *M. microti*, which cause tuberculosis, or *M. lepraemurium*, the cause of feline leprosy (see next chapter). In addition, various other mycobacteria may be involved in chronic wounds and abscesses.

EPIDEMIOLOGY

Tuberculosis is a rare disease of cats, but is slightly more common in dogs. *M. tuberculosis* and *M. bovis* infections are generally contracted from humans, although cattle and wild mammals might be an alternative source of infection in some areas. *M. avium* is a saprophyte found in soil and water, and only an opportunist pathogen of animals and man, while the main source of *M. microti* is probably voles: *M. avium* and *M. microti* infections are extremely rare.

CLINICAL SIGNS

- Generally acquired by respiratory, oral or percutaneous routes.
- Infection is usually subclinical.
- Clinical signs generally reflect the location of granulomas.
- In dogs, TB is usually respiratory, whereas in cats it is usually alimentary.
- Retching, a non-productive cough, dysphagia or hypersalivation reflect chronic ulceration of the oropharynx, tonsils and draining lymph nodes and bronchopneumonia.
- Anorexia, wasting, vomiting or diarrhoea may accompany intestinal malabsorption owing to granulomas in the alimentary tract, possibly with pleural or peritoneal effusion.
- Intestinal infection often causes palpably enlarged mesenteric lymph nodes.
- Skin and ocular forms can also occur in the cat.

DIAGNOSIS

- Usually based on a combination of history and the demonstration of acid-fast organisms in biopsies or smears of exudates.
- Isolation may be possible on special media, but can be a lengthy process.
- Radiography may reveal large granulomas in the respiratory tract or abdomen.
- Skin tests do not work in cats, and can be inconsistent in dogs.
- Very often diagnosis is made at necropsy.

TREATMENT

Improvement of clinical signs following treatment of cats with either isoniazid or streptomycin has been reported, but did not produce a bacteriological cure. Successful treatment of dogs experimentally infected with *M. tuberculosis* has been reported with rifampin, isoniazid and streptomycin for 23 months.

However, as bacteriological cure is rare, euthanasia is often recommended on public health grounds.

35 FELINE LEPROSY

AETIOLOGY

Feline leprosy is caused by *Mycobacterium lepraemurium* ('rat leprosy'). It is an uncommon condition thought to be contracted from rat (or other rodent) bites.

CLINICAL SIGNS

- Single or multiple, fleshy, sometimes ulcerated nodules on head or limbs.
- Lesions develop between 2 weeks and several months following injury.
- Spread of the infection up limb may be accompanied by lymphangitis and regional lymphadenopathy.

DIAGNOSIS

Diagnosis is based on finding acid-fast organisms in impression smears or biopsies. *M. lepraemurium* is very difficult to grow *in vitro*, so isolation is not usually attempted.

TREATMENT

The usual treatment is surgical removal.

Oral dapsone at 50 mg twice a day for 2 weeks may be worth trying. Haemolytic anaemia and neurotoxicity have been reported with dapsone in cats, so the canine dose rate of 1 mg/kg three times daily may be more appropriate.

Recurrence of lesions at the same or other sites often occurs.

36 ATYPICAL MYCOBACTERIAL INFECTIONS

Occasionally, in cats and dogs various saprophytic mycobacteria including the *M. fortuitum–M. chelonei* complex, *M. smegmatis*, *M. xenopi* and *M. phlei* have been isolated from:

- superficial or, rarely, deeper persistent abscesses;
- ulcerative lesions; or
- granulomatous lesions.

TREATMENT

Treatment is by surgical removal/drainage combined with antibiotics. Gentamicin (2 mg/kg IM or SC twice daily) or potentiated sulphonamides (10–15 mg/kg orally twice a day) are sometimes useful as the usual anti-tuberculous antibiotics are usually ineffective. Treatment is apparently more likely to be successful in dogs than in cats.

See also Chapter 35, Feline Leprosy.

37 STREPTOCOCCAL INFECTIONS

AETIOLOGY

Beta-haemolytic streptococci of Lancefield group G are part of the normal flora of the upper respiratory tract, oropharynx, lower genital tract and skin of cats and dogs. Most animals probably become infected at birth from the mother's genital tract. Infection enters through umbilicus then spreads around body via liver.

CLINICAL SIGNS

- In healthy puppies and kittens born of older dams, maternal antibody generally protects against clinical disease.
- In litters born of younger dams, or if the litter or their dam are immunocompromised, septicaemia and severe systemic disease, often culminating in death, may develop.
- In older kittens, up to 6 months old, subclinical infection in tonsils may develop into clinical tonsillitis and cervical lymphadenopathy.
- In addition, group B, C and G streptococci are frequently isolated from wounds and abscesses in adult cats and dogs and as opportunist pathogens secondary to upper respiratory and other mucosal infections.

TREATMENT AND CONTROL

Affected puppies and kittens can be very difficult to treat. Often, puppies and kittens will not suckle, and rapidly become weak and dehydrated.

Good nursing and rehydration with subcutaneous or intraperitoneal fluids is important, together with an injection of long-acting penicillins.

In colonies with a history of neonatal disease, topical antiseptics on the navel and treatment at birth with long-acting penicillin or a penicillin derivative may help prevent further disease.

PUBLIC HEALTH ASPECTS

Both cats and dogs can also harbour asymptomatic infections of group A streptococci in their oropharynx. Group A streptococci are more often associated with human disease. Hence the family pet may become a reservoir for human infection and the source of recurrent tonsillitis or pharyngitis in a family.

38 TYZZER'S DISEASE

AETIOLOGY

Tyzzer's disease is an uncommon disease of cats and dogs and is caused by *Clostridium piliformis. Cl. piliformis* is part of the normal intestinal flora of many rodents, but can cause clinical disease if the host is immunosuppressed in some way.

Cats and dogs are thought to become infected through contact with rodents, and may also be more susceptible to disease if immunosuppressed or under stress.

Cl. piliformis replicates inside intestinal epithelial cells, may cause iliocolitis and may spread to cause focal necrotic hepatitis.

CLINICAL SIGNS

- rapid onset anorexia;
- depression;
- abdominal pain and distension;
- hepatomegaly and, possibly, jaundice;
- death within 2 days.

DIAGNOSIS

Diagnosis is usually made post mortem, based on gross and microscopic lesions and isolation of *Cl. piliformis*.

39 COLIBACILLOSIS

Little is known about the role of *Escherichia coli* in canine and feline enteric disease. *E. coli* is part of the normal flora of the gut, but some studies suggest that certain cases of acute diarrhoea might be caused by *E. coli* capable of producing toxins related to those produced by enteropathogenic *E. coli* of other species.

E. coli can often be isolated from urine of healthy cats and dogs, although many such isolations probably reflect faecal contamination of the sample. High numbers ($>10^3$/ml urine), however, may be associated with pyelonephritis or acute cystitis.

E. coli is also frequently isolated from many sites and the blood of fading puppies and kittens, from abscesses, wounds and pyometra and from peritonitis following bowel injuries or rupture.

40 SALMONELLOSIS

The prevalence of *Salmonella* spp infection in dogs and cats is much higher than the incidence of clinical disease; amongst dogs, faecal surveys generally find 1–5% normal dogs and cats shedding *Salmonella* spp and it is more common (up to 25%) in puppies less than 6 months old.

Cats are extremely resistant to experimental infection with *Salmonella* spp, and clinical salmonellosis is uncommon in cats, although epizootics may occur, especially in kittens.

CLINICAL SALMONELLOSIS

- Usually associated, in both cats and dogs, with concurrent enteric infections or immunosuppression.
- Serotypes isolated are mostly *S. typhimurium*, but reflect local conditions and include whichever serotypes dominate at the time.
- Clinical syndromes include:

  - acute and chronic gastroenteritis
  - pyrexic episodes lasting several days
  - vomiting
  - pneumonia
  - conjunctivitis
  - abortion
  - stillbirths
  - fading puppies or kittens.

- Severe infection may result in:

  - bacteraemia
  - endotoxaemia
  - depression
  - hypothermia
  - collapse.

- Transient bacteraemias sometimes result in abscess formation in internal organs such as the liver, lung, spleen, lymph nodes or bone marrow.

TREATMENT

- Initially symptomatic.
- Avoid antibiotics whenever possible as they rarely eliminate the organism, may cause selection of resistant strains and may prolong shedding. Multi-resistant salmonellae have been isolated from cats.
- When antibacterial treatment is necessary, choose the antibiotic on basis of sensitivity test.

PUBLIC HEALTH ASPECTS

The source of infection in cats and dogs is often difficult to determine but is probably generally similar to that in humans, e.g. contaminated food, particularly meat products. An exception to this is salmonellosis in kittens acquired from hunting or scavenging wild birds. Although transmission to man is possible, a common source of infection is perhaps more likely when salmonellae are isolated from both owners and their cat or dog.

41 BOTULISM

Botulism is caused by ingestion of *Clostridium botulinum* toxin in water or food. Cats are very resistant to botulinum toxin, and feline botulism is therefore very rare.

In dogs, the severity of disease depends on the amount of toxin ingested.

CLINICAL SIGNS

Clinical signs include:

- flaccid paralysis in hind limbs;
- progressing forward to forelimbs;
- then paralysis of respiratory muscles leading to abdominal respiration; and
- possibly eventual death.
- May also see:
  - ○ megaoesophagus
  - ○ constipation
  - ○ urinary retention.

DIAGNOSIS

This relies on detection of toxin in serum, vomit or food.

TREATMENT

Treatment is supportive:

- catheterise bladder
- enemas
- fluids
- antibiotics to prevent secondary infections.

Antitoxin is not effective after toxin has entered nerves, so its use is controversial.

42 TETANUS

Tetanus is caused by the neurotoxin tetanospasmin, produced by the growth of *Clostridium tetani* in anaerobic conditions. Highly resistant spores are found in the soil; organisms can be routinely isolated from faeces of cats and dogs, but toxin produced in the gut is destroyed by digestion.

Dogs, and even more so cats, are relatively resistant to tetanus. Feline tetanus is a rare disease. Toxin produced in a wound travels up nerves, and gradually involves the whole CNS.

CLINICAL SIGNS

First sign is therefore often local spastic paralysis, e.g. of one limb. Gradually involves whole body. Affected animals have:

- stiff gait
- outstretched tail
- erect ears
- contraction of the facial muscles giving the animal a surprised look
- may be hyperaesthetic
- muscle spasms or convulsions
- dysuria
- drooling
- constipation.

In severe cases, respiratory paralysis leads to death.

DIAGNOSIS

Largely by clinical signs and history of wound.

TREATMENT

Treatment involves thorough debridement and cleansing of the wound, and administration of intravenous or intramuscular penicillin G (20 mg/kg twice daily) for at least 5 days.

Prompt therapy with antitoxin has been recommended intravenously (100–500 units/kg) or by local infiltration. However, as it does not penetrate the CNS the efficacy of this therapy is debatable and there also exists a risk of anaphylactic reactions to the antiserum.

Animals should be kept in a quiet and darkened room and disturbed as little as possible as they may be hyperaesthetic.

Barbiturate or phenothiazine group drugs may be helpful to control tetanic spasms. Diazepam (0.2 mg/kg IV as necessary) can be given for sedation.

General nursing care is also important to empty the bladder and rectum and to ensure adequate nutrition and hydration.

Nutritional support (enteral or parenteral) may be necessary.

43 LYME DISEASE/ BORRELIOSIS

AETIOLOGY

Borrelia burgdorferi is a spirochaete transmitted by *Ixodes* ticks, with its main reservoir in wild rodents and deer. It has recently been suggested that *B. burgdorferi* ought to be further divided into several different species with differing geographic distributions and virulence to man and domestic animals. This might help explain the apparently different clinical features of infection in North America and Europe.

Infection is fairly common in some parts of Britain such as Cumbria and the New Forest. In North America it is mainly found in the North-East USA. In North America the tick is believed to have a 2 year life cycle but in Europe the cycle may be 3 years.

There are no reports of dog-to-human transmission, so canine and feline infections should not be regarded as zoonotic.

CLINICAL SIGNS

- There may be a long incubation period as the bacterium can lie dormant in the host and only cause disease months or years after infection.
- However, most infected animals (including man) never develop any clinical signs.
- Clinical signs may include:

  ○ a rash
  ○ pyrexia
  ○ depression
  ○ persistent lymphadenopathy
  ○ chronic arthritis
  ○ chronic neurological disease.

DIAGNOSIS

Diagnosis is based on a combination of clinical signs and serology. Isolation of the spirochate is difficult and some laboratories use PCR to detect the organism.

It is very important not to confuse present or past infection, as detected by antibody tests, with evidence of disease. In Western Europe, at least, serological evidence of infection in cats and dogs is quite common in some areas – but clinical disease is extremely rare.

TREATMENT

Antibiotic therapy such as tetracycline (10–20 mg/kg orally three times daily for 2 weeks) or, if no response, penicillin G (22 mg/kg IV four times daily for 1 week).

In man, mild analgesics such as aspirin are recommended for arthritis, but the response to antibiotic therapy in dogs is apparently very rapid so such treatment is probably not necessary.

PREVENTION

This is largely based on avoiding areas where infected ticks are likely to be found. At the time of writing, there are no commercially available vaccines for use in animals, although several experimental vaccines appear to be effective at preventing infection.

44 FELINE RICKETTSIAL INFECTIONS

Q FEVER

AETIOLOGY

Q-fever is caused by *Coxiella burnetii*, a rickettsia. Although, like other rickettsiae, *C. burnetii* can be transmitted between and from ticks, *C. burnetii* can also be maintained in wild and domestic animal populations by ingestion and inhalation of infectious material such as placentas, urine and faeces.

CLINICAL SIGNS

- Antibody to Q-fever is apparently quite common in domestic cats; surveys in the the USA and UK suggest that up to 40% of cats may have been subclinically infected at some time.
- The role of *C. burnetii* in feline disease is not known, although it may be an occasional cause of abortion or premature parturition.
- The role of cats in the epidemiology of human infection is not known and requires further investigation.

TREATMENT

As infection in dogs and cats is often subclinical or is diagnosed only retrospectively, there is little information available on treatment. Tetracyclines, potentiated sulphonamides and quinalones have all been suggested.

PUBLIC HEALTH

Apart from occasional abortions in sheep and cattle, *C. burnetii* generally causes no disease in most of its hosts.

SECTION 4

The main exception is man, in whom infection can cause:

- general malaise
- pyrexia
- pneumonia
- myalgia
- vomiting and diarrhoea.

Traditionally, veterinary surgeons, abattoir workers and farmers were most at risk of infection, but more recently urban outbreaks have occurred in the UK where the source of infection was difficult to determine. In North America there have been several reports of Q fever in man contracted from parturient and aborting cats.

FELINE INFECTIOUS ANAEMIA (HAEMOBARTONELLOSIS)

AETIOLOGY

The rickettsia *Haemobartonella felis* adheres to cat red blood cells, damaging the cell surface and leading to removal of infected erythrocytes from the circulation by phagocytes in the spleen and liver.

The replication cycle takes 3–8 weeks, resulting in cyclical variations in bacteraemia and therefore also in clinical signs.

Dogs can be infected with *H. canis*, but this rarely causes clinical disease.

EPIDEMIOLOGY

- Route of transmission not known; probably requires blood transfer by, for example, fleas.
- Transmission from queens to kittens also occurs – but not known if this happens during pregancy, at birth or via milk.

CLINICAL SIGNS

Infection is often asymptomatic, and clinical disease may develop only when the cat suffers stress or is immunosuppressed, for example by feline leukaemia virus or feline immunodeficiency virus infections.

- Anaemia: pale mucous membranes, lethargy, tachypnoea, dyspnoea on exertion, tachycardia.
- Splenomegaly.

- Possibly pyrexia.
- Possibly haemic murmur if anaemia is very severe.
- Occasionally jaundice due to massive haemolysis.
- In addition to the anaemia caused directly by the infection, some infected cats also develop an immune-mediated haemolytic anaemia which further increases the loss of red blood cells.
- *H. felis* can also cause persistent infections, probably in the spleen. Persistently infected cats may become clinically asymptomatic carriers, probably for years, possibly for life.

DIAGNOSIS

Giemsa or acridine orange stained blood smears may reveal the organisms as small round dots (perhaps in chains), rings or rods, adherent to red blood cells.

Experience is required to accurately interpret smears, and, because of the cyclic nature of the infection, several samples taken over a period of several weeks may have to be examined to detect the organisms. *Note:* smears will almost certainly be negative for *H. felis* if antibiotics, particularly tetracyclines, have been given.

The anaemia is regenerative, with polychromasia and increased numbers of reticulocytes. Nucleated red blood cells may be present in smears. Spherocytes may be detected but should not be interpreted as evidence of regeneration in the absence of reticulocytosis.

TREATMENT

- Oxytetracycline (10–20 mg/kg orally three times daily) or doxycyline (5 mg/kg twice daily) for 3 weeks is fairly effective at controlling infection, but usually does not totally eliminate infection.
- In those cases where immune mediated haemolytic anaemia occurs, prednisolone (1–2 mg/kg orally twice daily) may be helpful. The dose should be reduced over 6–8 weeks depending on progress.
- Blood transfusions may be given in severe cases or fluid therapy may be required.

CAT SCRATCH DISEASE (CSD) AND BACILLARY ANGIOMATOSIS (BA)

AETIOLOGY

Until recently the cause(s) of CSD and BA were unknown. Recently, however, attention has been focused on two organisms, *Afipia felis* and *Bartonella henselae* (old name, *Rochalimaea henselae*). *A. felis* has only been isolated in a very few laboratories, whereas *B. henselae* (or sometimes the closely related *B. quintana*) is frequently isolated from cases of both CSD and BA in North America.

The incidence of CSD in Europe is not known. In the USA, estimates range from 6000 to over 20 000 cases each year, 2000 of which require hospitalization. A survey of cat blood samples from San Francisco for evidence of *B. henselae* bacteraemia reported *B. henselae* in 25 out of 61 cats (41%). The authors have been unable to detect *B. henselae* by isolation or PCR in blood from just over 20 British cats.

Transmission of *B. henselae* between cats or cats and humans may be via cat fleas. *A. felis*, however, is probably acquired from the environment, particularly soil.

CLINICAL SIGNS

Cat scratch disease and bacillary angiomatosis are human diseases.

A. felis and *B. henselae* appear to cause no known disease in cats, although longer term studies suggested that cats can remain bacteraemic for at least 17 months.

Cat scratch disease

- Generally a benign, self-limiting disease, usually seen in children.
- Almost all patients with CSD have had contact with a cat or dog but around 30% have no apparent history of a cat scratch.
- Primary skin lesion, usually at the site of a recent scratch or wound
  - first appears as a non-pruritic, erythematous papule;
  - develops into a vesicle, then pustule;
  - which ruptures, scabs over and heals.

- Regional lymphadenitis develops about a week after the skin lesion and may last several months.
- By the time the patient seeks medical help, lymphadenitis is often the only clinical sign.
- Atypical CSD (5–10% cases) includes:
  - Perinaud's oculoglandular syndrome (after conjunctival inoculation);
  - encephalitis (especially in adults);
  - recurrent or suppurative lymphadenitis;
  - retinitis;

○ arthralgia/arthritis;
○ systemic lesions (e.g. in the spleen).

● Bacillary angiomatosis is a disease mainly associated with HIV infection and characterised by multiple subcutaneous nodules.

DIAGNOSIS

Histology

Examination of lymph nodes from CSD cases reveals focal necrosis, vascular proliferation and clumps of extracellular, pleomorphic bacilli visible only with special silver stains.

In BA, proliferation of small blood vessels with variable necrosis and neutrophil invasion is seen in skin lesions and often also in underlying bone marrow, lymph nodes and major organs such as spleen and liver.

Detection of *Bartonella* spp or *A. felis*

Both organisms can be difficult to grow, but under the appropriate conditions will grow slowly either on special bacterial media or in some cell cultures. More rapid identification of *Bartonella* spp can be made by use of a polymerase chain reaction on lesion material from human cases or blood of cats.

TREATMENT

Antibiotic therapy of human CSD and BA has not generally proved useful, although some workers have had some success with intravenous gentamicin in severe cases.

B. henselae appeared to be eliminated from three cats treated with either doxycycline (25–50 mg twice daily, orally) or lincomycin (100 mg twice daily, orally).

SECTION 4

45 CANINE RICKETTSIAL INFECTIONS

SALMON POISONING DISEASE AND ELOKOMIN FLUKE FEVER

Salmon poisoning disease (SPD) is caused by *Neorickettsia helminthoeca* and Elokomin fluke fever (EFF) by *N. elokominica*, two rickettsias transmitted by a trematode vector *Nanophytus salmonica*. The trematode harbours the rickettsias throughout its life cycle, which is complex and involves two intermediate hosts, a snail and salmonid fish; the adult fluke is found in fish-eating mammals and birds. The disease is seen mainly on the west coast of North America, coincident with the distribution of the snail intermediate host (*Oxytrema silicula*). Although the fluke has a fairly wide host range, rickettsial disease is generally seen only in dogs: cats are not susceptible.

CLINICAL SIGNS

SPD has a high mortality whereas EFF generally causes less severe disease. Both are characterised by:

- pyrexia
- followed by hypothermia
- depression
- anorexia
- diarrhoea and vomiting
- anaemia
- extreme weight loss.

In SPD, death often occurs within 10 days of the onset of clinical signs.

DIAGNOSIS

- Demonstration of fluke eggs in faeces.
- Cytology of lymph node aspirates.

TREATMENT

Parenteral oxytetracycline (10 mg/kg) for at least 3–5 days.

Symptomatic: fluids, anti-emetics, fasting to relieve diarrhoea; praziquantel (10–30 mg/kg, subcutaneous or oral) to eliminate fluke infection.

CANINE EHRLICHIOSIS

Caused by *Ehrlichia canis*, and transmitted by ticks (*Rhipicephalus sanguineus*), canine ehrlichiosis is seen in the Americas, Africa, Asia and southern Europe.

- Acute phase of the disease is often mild, but may be accompanied by depression, anorexia and pyrexia.
- Dogs may eliminate infection after the acute phase or go on to develop chronic infection which may last several years.
- Chronically infected dogs often appear clinically healthy, but some develop:

  ○ severe depression
  ○ weight loss
  ○ anaemia (due to decreased platelet survival)
  ○ episodic haemorrhage
  ○ and may die.

Diagnosis is based on finding ticks during the acute phase, haematology including demonstration of rickettsia in mononuclear cells or neutrophils, and serology.

Treatment is with oxytetracycline (22 mg/kg three times daily for 2–3 weeks) or doxycycline (5–10 mg/kg twice daily for one week.)

INFECTIOUS CYCLIC THROMBOCYTOPENIA (ICT)

Caused by *Ehrlichia platys* and transmitted by ticks, ICT is seen mainly in the southern USA and southern Europe. Cycles of parasitaemia and thrombocytopenia at 1 to 2 week intervals may cause:

- mild anaemia
- occasional haemorrhage
- pyrexia and depression

but usually cause no clinical disease.

SECTION 4

Diagnosis is by blood smears (rickettsia seen in platelets) and serology. Treatment is with tetracycline or doxycycline.

ROCKY MOUNTAIN SPOTTED FEVER (RMSF)

Caused by *Rickettsia rickettsia* and transmitted by *Dermacentor* spp ticks, RMSF is found throughout the Americas. *R. rickettsia* replicates in vascular endothelium and can cause multi-systemic severe disease in both man and dogs. Clinical signs include:

- fever
- cutaneous oedema
- arthralgia/myalgia
- neurological signs
- lymphadenopathy
- haemorrhage
- death.

Diagnosis is by haematology, direct immunofluorescence of infected tissues (store tissues in normal saline on ice), isolation of the organism at specialist laboratories, and serology.

Treatment is with oxytetracycline (22 mg/kg three times daily for up to 2 weeks) or doxycycline (10 mg/kg twice daily for 1 week).

46 OTHER BACTERIAL INFECTIONS

LISTERIOSIS

Listeria monocytogenes is a rare cause of disease in cats and dogs. Following ingestion, septicaemia and widespread microabscess formation can occur, causing signs related to the organs most affected.

ANTHRAX

Bacillus anthracis infection is very rare in dogs and cats. Clinical signs include severe local inflammation and necrosis of the upper alimentary tract, head and neck. Anthrax is a notifiable disease.

Anaerobiospirillum spp INFECTION

Anaerobiospirillum spp are fairly recently described spiral bacteria which have been isolated from the faeces of children with diarrhoea but not from normal human faeces. However, *Anaerobiospirillum* spp is a normal finding in cat and dog faeces, and transmission from a puppy to a baby has been reported.

STAPHYLOCOCCAL INFECTIONS

Although canine isolates have been shown experimentally to grow on human skin, and vice versa, there is little evidence that transmission occurs in the field.

However, there are some reports of non-phage-typable apparent *Staphylococcus aureus* isolates from humans turning out to be *Staphylococcus intermedius*, which is normally found on animals, particularly dogs, so the possibility of zoonotic spread exists.

YERSINIOSIS

AETIOLOGY

Yersinia enterocolitica and *Y. pseudotuberculosis* can be isolated from the soil and from faeces of many animals, including cats and dogs.

CLINICAL SIGNS

- Generally cause no clinical signs in cats and dogs.
- But *Y. enterocolitica* has been associated with mild gastroenteritis in puppies.
- *Y. pseudotuberculosis* can cause gastroenteritis, abdominal lymphadenitis and multiple caseous abscesses in liver, kidneys and spleen.
- In man, particularly young children, both can cause severe disease.

TREATMENT AND CONTROL

If a cat or dog is shown to be shedding *Y. enterocolitica* or *Y. pseudotuberculosis* in its faeces, then treatment with tetracyclines or potentiated sulphonamides may be thought appropriate.

PLAGUE

In some parts of North America, cats can become infected with the plague organism, *Yersinia pestis*, through contact with wild mammals or their fleas. They may pass the infection on to man, veterinary surgeons being particularly at risk.

The prevalence of infection in European wildlife is not known but is probably low, and the risk of feline (and human) infection in Europe is therefore probably small.

The most common form of the disease in cats is bubonic plague, clinical signs of which include pyrexia, dehydration and lymphadenopathy.

Septicaemic plague is often fatal within several days with few signs other than collapse and shock. Pneumonic plague is rare in cats.

Treatment is by drainage and lavage of buboes and intramuscular amino-glycoside injections (streptomycin at 5 mg/kg twice daily or gentamicin at 2 mg/kg twice daily) for 3 weeks.

Capnocytophaga canimorsus and *C. cynodegmi* INFECTIONS

Also known as dysgonic fermenter type 2 (DF-2) and DF-2-like organisms.

Part of the normal flora of many animal species' mouths, particularly dogs and cats, these pleomorphic Gram-negative bacteria are commonly transmitted through bites and scratches but usually cause no or little disease in man. However, in immunosuppressed and splenoctomised individuals, they can cause severe disease including septicaemia, septic endocarditis, arthritis, meningoencephalitis and death. It can take up to 10 days to detect *Capnocytophaga* spp in culture, so treatment is usually begun as soon as infection is suspected. Although most isolates are susceptible to penicillin, some are not, leading to further delays in onset of effective treatment.

SOME OTHER BACTERIA ASSOCIATED WITH DOG AND CAT BITE WOUNDS IN MAN

Pasteurella spp. The most commonly isolated organisms from human wounds caused by cat (up to 75%) or dog (up to 38%) bites. Can cause severe systemic infections in man.

Eikenella corrodens. A Gram-negative capnophilic rod, found in gingival plaque from around 60% of dogs (and man). An increasingly frequent isolate from dog-bite wounds in man.

Pseudomonas spp, *Actinobacillus* spp, streptococci, staphylococci, *Corynebacterium* spp, and a variety of anaerobes are also commonly isolated from human wounds caused by cat or dog bites.

SECTION 4

Helicobacter INFECTIONS

Helicobacter-like organisms have been isolated from the stomach of both cats and dogs. However, the clinical and zoonotic implications of this are unclear.

EUGONIC FERMENTER TYPE 4

- EF-4 is a Gram-negative bacterium, with cultural properties similar to those of *Pasteurella* spp.
- Part of the normal commensal flora of the oral cavity of cats and dogs and many other carnivores, possibly including badgers.
- Isolated from purulent bite wounds, otitis, sinusitis, focal necrotic pneumonia, and septicaemia in animals and man.
- EF-4 has also been associated with fatal pneumonia in cats, causing sudden death.
- Recent transportation or other stresses may be predisposing factors.

TULARAEMIA

Caused by *Francisella tularensis*, a Gram-negative pleomorphic rod, enzootic in wild rabbits and rodents among which it is transmitted by various ticks. Type A is found in North America and is the more virulent form, whereas type B rarely causes disease in any host and occurs in the rest of the Northern hemisphere.

- Cats and dogs usually become infected either by tick bites or by ingestion of infected rabbits or contaminated water.
- Clinical signs in dogs are rare and usually mild.
- In cats clinical signs include:

  ○ depression, anorexia and pyrexia
  ○ lymphadenopathy, splenomegaly, hepatomegaly
  ○ oral and tongue ulceration
  ○ abscesses
  ○ jaundice.

- Cat-to-man transmission has been reported. Clinical signs in man are similar to those in the cat.

Diagnosis is by isolation of *F. tularensis* at specialist laboratories. Treatment of cats and dogs is rarely successful.

Section 5
FUNGAL, ALGAL AND PROTOZOAL INFECTIONS

47 DERMATOPHYTOSIS (RINGWORM)

AETIOLOGY

Although many dermatophytes have been isolated from skin lesions of cats and dogs, by far the majority of cases are caused by *Microsporum canis* (probably >90% of feline cases and approximately 50–70% of canine cases). The remainder are usually caused by *Trichophyton mentagrophytes* and *M. gypseum*.

EPIDEMIOLOGY

The source of most dermatophyte infections is other animals. *M. canis* infections in both cats and dogs usually originate from contact with an infected cat, whereas many *T. mentagrophytes* infections are thought to originate from rodents. *M. gypseum*, however, is a soil organism.

The arthrospores of dermatophytes are, however, very resistant, and can survive in the environment, on furniture and equipment, for several years, providing a long-term source of infection.

CLINICAL SIGNS

The clinical signs of dermatophytosis are very variable in both cats and dogs, and a diagnosis cannot be made on clinical signs alone. A history of contact with other infected animals or lesions on in-contact humans can be helpful.

Cats

Clinical signs may be mild and difficult to find. Many authors believe that non-symptomatic carriage is common in cats, especially in longhair breeds, but others suggest that most infected cats do have some clinical signs if a thorough examination is carried out.

Most frequently, clinical signs of feline dermatophytosis consist of irregular patches of hair loss, sometimes with some skin scaling.

SECTION 5

However, may also see:

- granulomatous lesions
- miliary dermatitis
- onychomycosis
- or 'typical' circular patches of alopecia with scaling.

More severe clinical signs are seen particularly in young kittens or cats which are in some way immunosuppressed, malnourished or have a pre-existing skin condition.

Dogs

Ringworm is far less common in dogs than it is in cats, and dogs often develop the classical circular areas of alopecia and scaling. However, the same range of lesions as seen in cats can also be found in dogs.

DIAGNOSIS

- Many cases of *M. canis* infection fluoresce apple green when illuminated with a Wood's lamp (ultra-violet light, 365–366 nm). However, this technique requires some experience to be interpreted correctly, and obviously will not detect all cases of dermatophytosis.
- Hairs plucked from the periphery of a lesion can be examined by direct light microscopy, after incubation in 10% potassium hydroxide, for chains of arthrospores along hair shafts or in attached scale material. However, this technique also requires some experience if its results are to be interpreted correctly.
- Definitive diagnosis depends on culture in Sabaraud dextrose agar or Dermatophyte Test Medium (DTM) and identification of any organisms which grow, by colony morphology and microscopic examination of their spore-producing macroconidia.
- Samples for culture may be plucked hairs and scrapings from the edge of lesions. The lesions should first be clipped and then patted with an ethanol-soaked swab to reduce bacterial contamination. For animals without clinical signs, careful brushings taken with a sterile toothbrush (soak in 0.1% chlorhexidine solution for 30 minutes) are ideal; the bristles are directly pressed in to the agar.

TREATMENT

Dermatophytosis is often a self-limiting disease, with recovery within a few months, so clipping and topical therapy may be all that is required in many cases – especially since systemic therapy may be accompanied by side effects.

- Ideally the animal should have all its hair clipped, but, if this is not possible, then the areas around all lesions must be clipped.
- Clippings should be disposed of carefully as they may be infectious to man.
- Infected areas should be bathed to remove scale, crusts or exudate and treated topically, for example with daily whole-body baths in povidone iodine or chlorhexidine.

In severe or chronic cases, the treatment of choice is oral griseofulvin. The dose usually recommended for microsized formulations is 15–20 mg/kg/day in cats, although some authors suggest higher doses of up to 150 mg/kg/day for both cats and dogs. Griseofulvin treatment should be continued until at least 2 weeks after clinical recovery and until dermatophytes can no longer be isolated.

Note:

- Griseofulvin is teratogenic and therefore is contraindicated in pregnant animals.
- Other side effects of griseofulvin include vomiting, diarrhoea, anorexia, jaundice, anaemia, ataxia and depression.

Ketoconazole can be effective at treating dermatophyte infections, but also has side effects, is relatively expensive, and is not licensed for use in cats in the UK.

CONTROL

In-contact animals should be tested, and, if found to be infected, separated from those not infected and treated as above. In colonies of cats, uninfected in-contact cats may also be treated with griseofulvin for 2 weeks.

As dermatophytes can survive so well in the environment, environmental control is very important. Contaminated hair clippings, and disposable equipment and bedding etc. should be destroyed. Fixed elements of the environment should be vacuum cleaned and disinfected weekly with iodine, formalin or hypochlorite solutions.

Vaccines have been developed and licensed for use in other species, but more work is needed on their efficacy in cats.

PUBLIC HEALTH ASPECTS

The dermatophytes of cats and dogs are infectious to man, and cats are a frequent source of human ringworm, particularly to small children.

48 ASPERGILLOSIS

AETIOLOGY

Aspergillus spp are commonly found in the environment. The most common species to infect cats and dogs is *A. fumigatus* although other species may be involved.

CLINICAL SIGNS

Canine nasal aspergillosis

- bloody, purulent nasal discharge;
- ulceration of external nares, and nasal and facial pain;
- disseminated aspergillosis in dogs is extremely rare.

Feline aspergillosis

This is far less common than infection of dogs. Although it can cause chronic nasal disease, feline aspergillosis appears to be more often a systemic infection, causing granulomatous pneumonia or infiltrative intestinal lesions. As in other species, aspergillosis in the cat is usually associated with immunosuppression.

DIAGNOSIS

Diagnosis can be difficult.

- Culture and cytology may be unsuccessful, yet 40% of normal dogs may be positive.
- Histology of biopsies obtained blind from dogs is rather hit and miss.
- A combination of radiology (loss of turbinate structure), rhinoscopy (using a bronchoscope, or even an otoscope) and serology is most useful in dogs.
- Diagnosis in cats is often only made post mortem.

THERAPY

Nasal aspergillosis in dogs

- Topical enilconazole (10 mg/kg – dilute stock 10% solution with water to make emulsion, then use immediately) given twice daily for 1 week through tubes surgically implanted into the frontal sinuses.

Feline systemic aspergillosis

Treatment is possible, but is usually unsuccessful and the prognosis is poor. Possibly try:

- Amphotericin and 5-fluorocytosine.
- Thiabendazole or ketoconazole may also be effective.

49   CANDIDIASIS

AETIOLOGY

- *Candida albicans* is commonly isolated from the ears, nose, oral cavity and anus of dogs.
- May be an opportunist pathogen in immunosuppressed dogs or in chronic, non-healing ulcerative lesions (e.g. in chronic otitis externa).
- Rare pathogen of the cat – normally immunosuppressed or debilitated.

CLINICAL SIGNS

- Lesions are typically greyish mucoid plaques with a foul-smelling odour.
- Systemic and intestinal candidiasis, causing chronic diarrhoea, also occasionally occur.

DIAGNOSIS

Yeast-like organism can be seen in stained smears of lesions and biopsy material, and colonies rapidly grow on Sabaraud's agar.

THERAPY

Topical therapy with gentian violet or nystatin has been recommended, and systemic ketoconazole (5–10 mg/kg orally two or three times daily) may be used.
   The predisposing cause should, if possible, be treated.

50 OTHER FUNGAL INFECTIONS

BLASTOMYCOSIS

This infection, caused by the soil saprophyte *Blastomyces dermatitidis*, is mainly seen in North America. It can cause cutaneous, pulmonary or disseminated disease.

The site and severity of the lesions determine the clinical signs seen, although around a half of all affected dogs have cutaneous (ulcerated, sometimes granulomatous, nodules) and ocular (uveitis, glaucoma, retinal detachment) signs.

Diagnosis is usually by identification of yeast-like organisms in smears or thin sections of lesions.

Treatment is with amphotericin B (0.5 mg/kg in dogs, 0.25 mg/kg in cats, IV three times per week for several weeks or until biochemical evidence of renal dysfunction) sometimes followed by ketoconazole (10 mg/kg orally twice daily for up to two months).

HISTOPLASMOSIS

Found in soil world-wide, *Histoplasma capsulatum* infections are mainly a clinical problem in North America.

Causes pulmonary and systemic disease in cats, but in dogs the clinical signs are more often associated with systemic and gastrointestinal infection.

Diagnosis is usually by cytology of smears or histopathological examination.

Treatment is with ketoconazole (10–15 mg/kg orally twice daily for 4–6 months).

CRYPTOCOCCOSIS

Cryptococcosis occurs world-wide and has been reported, but is rarely diagnosed, in Britain. *Cryptococcus neoformans* is frequently associated with pigeon droppings. In man, infection is associated with immunosuppression and this may also be the case in the domestic cats and dogs.

Many organ systems can be involved, but the upper respiratory tract is the most common site of infection in cats, while in dogs neurological signs associated with CNS infection are most common.

Diagnosis is based on demonstration of the organism from lesions, or detection of antigen in sera.

Treatment can be attempted with ketoconazole or a combination of amphotericin B and 5-fluorocytosine, but the prognosis is always guarded.

COCCIDIOMYCOSIS

Coccidioides immitis is a soil saprophyte found mainly in desert areas of the south-western USA.

It can cause a kennel-cough-like syndrome in dogs.

Feline infection is very rare: in cat generally see skin lesions, possibly with respiratory signs.

Diagnosis is by serology and culture.

Treatment of choice is long-term ketoconazole (5–10 mg/kg orally twice daily for up to a year, then maintenance at 2–5 mg/kg daily to prevent relapses).

SPOROTRICHOSIS

Caused by inoculation of *Sporothrix schenckii* into the skin on thorns or other plant material.

Ulcerating dermal or subcutaneous nodules develop, often spreading along lymphatic vessels. Lesions on the faces of cats look like cat-bite abscesses. Necropsy often reveals systemic lymphatic spread to many internal organs.

Diagnosis is by cytology, histopathology and fungal culture.

Therapy in dogs is by giving supersaturated potassium iodide (40 mg kg orally three times daily) with food, or with ketoconazole (15 mg/kg orally twice daily), for 1 month beyond clinical cure. Treatment for cats is similar (but at around half the canine dose of potassium iodide or ketoconazole), but they must be carefully monitored for signs of iodism or ketoconazole toxicity.

RHINOSPORIDIOSIS

Rhinosporidium seeberi is found mainly in the Indian sub-continent and South America, but occurs sporadically world-wide.

The usual clinical signs are sneezing and a nasal discharge caused by the development of a unilateral polyp-like mass in the nares of large breeds of dog.

Diagnosis is by cytology and histopathology.

Treatment is surgical removal.

TRICHOSPOROSIS

Trichosporon spp are saprophytes found in the soil and as part of the normal skin and mucosal flora of many animals. Disease is thought to be secondary to immunosuppression or primary damage to skin or mucosae.

Trichosporosis is a rare cause of disease in cats; clinical signs usually consist of suppurative or granulomatous lesions of mucosae or subcutanous tissues.

Diagnosis is based on culture and demonstration of the organism in lesions by histopathology.

Treatment is with ketoconazole.

SECTION 5

51 PROTOTHECOSIS

AETIOLOGY

- *Prototheca* is a genus of algae, several species of which can be pathogenic to the dog and cat.
- It is found mainly in sewage, from which it can contaminate drinking water, soil and food.
- Animal-to-animal spread does not occur.
- Infection is most often seen in animals which are immunosuppressed, and is especially associated with depression of cell-mediated immunity.

CLINICAL SIGNS

- Dogs usually develop systemic infection with clinical signs which include:

  ○ intermittent, chronic, bloody diarrhoea
  ○ weight loss
  ○ signs of CNS and eye infection.

- Cats may develop systemic disease, but generally develop cutaneous nodules on the head or feet.

DIAGNOSIS

Diagnosis depends on demonstration of the organism in biopsies or in smears of vitreous fluid, CSF or, sometimes, urine.
  Prototheca will grow in Sabaraud's media.

TREATMENT

- Treatment of skin lesions in cats is surgical excision.
- There is no known effective treatment for systemic infection.

52 TOXOPLASMOSIS

AETIOLOGY

- Caused by protozoan, *Toxoplasma gondii*.
- Wide host range.

PATHOGENESIS (Figure 52.1)

- Sexual reproduction of *T. gondii* apparently occurs only in cats. After the cat ingests a tissue cyst in food, the cyst breaks down to release bradyzoites which reproduce in the wall of the intestine, eventually giving rise to oocysts which are passed out in the faeces.
- The oocyst further develops for 24 hours or more (depending on environmental temperature) before infectious sporozoites form.
- Only sporulated oocysts are infectious.
- Ingestion of sporulated oocysts by an intermediate host (e.g. rodent, dog, man or sheep) leads to release of sporozoites which penetrate the intestinal wall, multiply asexually as tachyzoites, become widely disseminated and encyst in tissues.
- The cycle is completed when a cat eats cysts in an intermediate host.
- Toxoplasmosis can also be transmitted between non-feline hosts if one eats the other (e.g. dog or man eating infected sheep meat).
- There is also some evidence that transplacental transmission of tissue cysts may occur in some rodent species.
- Most cats become infected by ingestion of tissue cysts in prey (e.g. rodents) or other food (raw meat). Shedding of oocysts in faeces is most common in kittens, but can occur in any age of cat (and may be enhanced by, for example, feline immunodeficiency virus infection).
- Oocysts can remain infectious for several months and are quite resistant to disinfectants, drying and freezing. Tissue cysts are less resistant, and are destroyed by proper cooking of food.

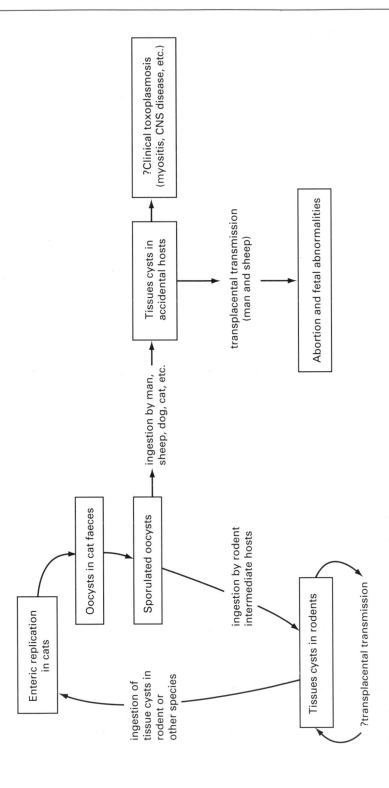

Figure 52.1 The pathogenesis of toxoplasmosis

CLINICAL SIGNS

Cats

- Replication in the gut is usually asymptomatic, but may rarely cause mild diarrhoea.
- Tissue cysts of *T. gondii* usually cause no clinical signs in cats. If they do, clinical signs reflect the major organs involved and include:

  ○ anorexia and depression
  ○ dyspnoea
  ○ ocular lesions such as uveitis and keratic precipitates
  ○ possibly jaundice, vomiting, diarrhoea
  ○ pyrexia
  ○ neurological signs.

- Congenital infection of kittens is a rare cause of fading kitten syndrome.

Dogs

- Usually asymptomatic.
- Clinical disease may be associated with stress and immunosuppression, such as distemper infection or corticosteroid treatment.

Clinical signs depend on the precise site of the lesion(s), and include:

- Neurological signs with lesions in the brain or spinal cord:

  ○ fits and tremors
  ○ ataxia
  ○ paralysis.

- Toxoplasmal myositis:

  ○ abnormal gait
  ○ muscle atrophy
  ○ stiffness.

- Severe disease and often rapidly fatal pneumonia or hepatitis.
- Myocardial infection.
- Ocular involvement is not so common in the dog as in the cat.

Infection in other hosts including man

Intermediate hosts (which may be virtually any mammal) may be infected either by eating cysts or oocysts: vertical transmission may also occur in some rodents.

Humans become infected through contact with infected cat faeces or through eating raw or undercooked meat.

SECTION 5

The formation of tissue cysts in the non-pregnant animal (or man) is usually not associated with the development of disease, though immunocompromised or elderly individuals may show clinical signs.

Infection of pregnant sheep causes abortion and birth of weakly lambs.

Infection of pregnant women can cause congenital infection and abnormalities of development in the fetus.

DIAGNOSIS

Antibody tests are available, but may not be particularly helpful in diagnosis of clinical disease as a positive test only indicates prior exposure, and around 40% of domestic cats are antibody positive. Paired serum samples, to demonstrate a rising titre, or IgM-specific assays may be more helpful.

Histopathological examination of tissues, including cerebrospinal fluid, and demonstration of tachyzoites may also assist in the diagnosis of clinical disease.

But, a diagnosis of toxoplasmosis is often only made at post-mortem examination, when the findings include pneumonia, hepatitis and mesenteric lymphadenopathy.

TREATMENT

If diagnosed in life, therapy may be attempted with:

- sulphonamides (30 mg/kg twice daily) in combination with pyrimethamine (0.5 mg/kg twice daily); or
- clindamycin (10 mg/kg twice daily).

However, the efficacy of therapy has not yet been accurately assessed.

CONTROL

Control of disease in cats can be attempted by feeding only dried, canned or cooked food.

Control of disease in sheep mainly relies on limiting exposure to infectious cat faeces or ensuring exposure is made when the sheep are not pregnant. Vaccines are now available for use in sheep.

Recommendations for the prevention of zoonotic spread include the following:

- Wear gloves to empty litter tray. This should be done daily, and the tray disinfected to remove all of faeces.
- Wear gloves while gardening or doing any other work which may lead to contact with material contaminated with cat faeces.
- Wash vegetables, especially home-grown, thoroughly.
- Wash hands thoroughly after handling raw meat.

- Cook meat thoroughly before consumption, and do not taste dishes during preparation.

Pregnant women should be especially careful and avoid emptying litter trays. A blood test prior to pregnancy can establish if the woman has already encountered the infection and therefore whether or not she is susceptible.

53 OTHER PROTOZOAL INFECTIONS

GIARDIASIS

Giardia duodenalis is a possible cause of acute and chronic diarrhoea in both puppies and kittens, but infections are often asymptomatic.

- Diagnosis is by identification of characteristic flagellated organisms in faeces.
- Treatment for 1 week with metronidazole (up to 30 mg/kg orally twice daily in dogs: 8–10 mg/kg orally twice daily in cats) or furazolidone (4 mg/kg orally twice daily) may be useful, but treatment often fails.

Although dogs and cats may be a source of human infection, infection from the same source (e.g. contaminated water supply) is more likely.

COCCIDIOSIS

Most frequently associated with *Isospora* spp in cats and dogs. Although sometimes associated with diarrhoea, *Isospora* spp infections are normally asymptomatic, and co-infection with other enteric pathogens or immunosuppression should be suspected if diarrhoea is seen. Potentiated sulphonamides (15 mg/kg orally three times daily) are probably the first line of treatment.

CRYPTOSPORIDIOSIS

Uncommon cause of mild diarrhoea in puppies and kittens. Be aware of the zoonotic risk – but cats and dogs probably infected from same source as man (e.g. contaminated water supply). Diagnosis is by use of special stains on faecal smears or sucrose flotation. There is no known effective treatment.

NEOSPOROSIS

Neospora caninum infection produces similar lesions and clinical signs to neuromuscular toxoplasmosis in dogs. Differentiation from toxoplasmosis is often made post mortem. There is no known treatment.

Pneumocystis carinii INFECTION

A protozoan found in the lungs of rats and humans, which can also infect cats and dogs. The significance of cat and dog infection is not known. In humans *P. carinii* generally causes no disease, although it is a common cause of pneumonia and death in AIDS sufferers.

LEISHMANIASIS

Canine leishmaniasis (feline infection is very rare) is most common in Mediterranean and South American countries, although occasional cases are also seen in Northern Europe and the southern USA. The protozoan is spread by biting sandflies.

Clinical signs in dogs include:

- skin lesions
- general debilitation due to infection of the major abdominal organs and immune complex formation
- terminal renal failure.

Diagnosis depends on identification of amastigotes in lymph-node or bone-marrow aspirates, special culture or (less sensitive) serology.

Treatment (meglumine antimonate 100 mg/kg or sodium stibogluconate 50 mg/kg daily) rarely eliminates the organism; relapses are common.

Dogs are an important reservoir of infection in the Mediterranean region, and, via sandflies, can be a source of human infection. Direct dog-to-human transmission can also occur, but is very rare.

HEPATOZOONOSIS

Canine *Hepatozoon canis* infection is found mainly in Africa, southern Europe and the southern USA. It is spread by ingestion of *Rhipicephalus* ticks. The clinical signs include pyrexia, weight loss, hind-limb and back pain and ocular and nasal discharge. Diagnosis is by identification of the parasite in blood smears. There is no effective treatment.

BABESIOSIS

Found world-wide (although very rare in UK), *Babesia* spp are spread by *Ixodes* ticks. Clinical signs depend on the age of dog (young animals are more susceptible) and the species and strain of parasite; they range from hyperacute haemolytic anaemia, shock and death, to acute haemolytic anaemia with haematuria and jaundice, and chronic weight loss. Parasites can be seen within erythrocytes. Treatments include diminazene aceturate (15 mg/kg, two subcutaneous injections given 24 hours apart), imidocarb diproprionate (6 mg/kg, subcutaneous or intramuscular) or intravenous trypan blue (10 mg/kg as 1% solution).

TRYPANOSOMIASIS

Chagas' disease, caused by *Trypanosoma cruzi*, is seen mainly in South and Central America and the southern USA. Infection is by ingestion of a reservoir host (e.g. opossums, raccoons, skunks) or from a reduviid vector ('kissing bug') bite. Clinical signs include depression, lymphadenopathy, cardiac failure and neurological disease. Diagnosis is by identification of trypanosomes in blood or lymph node aspirates, serology or culture. No effective treatment in dogs.

ENCEPHALITOZOONOSIS

Occasional infection of dogs and cats (and other carnivores such as mink) through contact with or ingestion of wild carnivores and rabbits. A possible cause of fading puppies, neurological signs and renal failure. The organisms can be detected in urine of affected animals. There is no treatment.

VACCINATION

Details of vaccination protocols for individual diseases are given (under 'Control') in the main text. This short chapter deals with some of the basic principles of vaccination of cats and dogs and with apparent vaccine failures and reactions.

CAT VACCINES AVAILABLE

Vaccine	Type	Route	See page
Feline panleucopenia	live or inact.	SC	35
Cat 'flu			
Feline herpesvirus	live	SC or IN	16
Feline calicivirus	live	SC or IN	16
Feline herpesvirus	inact.	SC	16
Feline calicivirus	inact.	SC	16
Feline leukaemia virus	inact. or recombinant	SC	53
Chlamydia psittaci felis	live	SC	25
Feline infectious peritonitis[1]	live	IN	45
Rabies	inact.	SC	101

DOG VACCINES AVAILABLE

Vaccine	Type	Route	See page
Canine distemper	live	SC	87
Canine parvovirus	live or inact.	SC	80
Infectious canine hepatitis[2]	live or inact.	SC	84
Leptospirosis			
interrogans icterohaemorrhagiae			
and L. interrogans canicola	inact.	SC	109
Kennel cough			
Canine parainfluenza	live	SC or IN[1]	94
Bordetella bronchiseptica	live	IN	93
Canine coronavirus[1]	live or inact.	SC	81
Rabies	live or inact.	SC	101

inact. = inactivated; SC = subcutaneous injection; IN = intranasal.
[1] Not available in the UK at the time of writing.
[2] Live vaccine is canine adenovirus (CAV) type 2 which protects against both CAV-1 (hepatitis) and CAV-2 (laryngotracheitis).

ROUTINE VACCINATION PROGRAMMES

Which vaccines are given and precisely when varies between countries and according to local factors such as disease prevalence and husbandry system (e.g. individual animal or colony).

Generally, routine vaccination is undertaken in puppies and kittens, with booster vaccination every one or two years depending on the vaccine.

Always read the manufacturer's recommendations, and consult with the manufacturer before deviating from their instructions.

Vaccination of puppies and kittens

- Aim is to provide active, vaccine-derived immunity as early as possible.
- But maternally derived antibody (MDA) may block effective vaccination in young animals. As MDA declines, they may become susceptible to infection before they are responsive to vaccination, leaving an 'immunity gap' (Figure 1). Some vaccines are better at overcoming MDA than others.
- In most diseases MDA declines to non-interfering levels in the majority of cats and dogs by 9–12 weks of age. The standard protocol is often therefore to vaccinate at 8 or 9 weeks and then repeat at 12 weeks old.
- Where puppies and kittens can be kept isolated and the risk of infection is low, one vaccine dose at 12 weeks of age will often suffice, particularly for modified live vaccines.

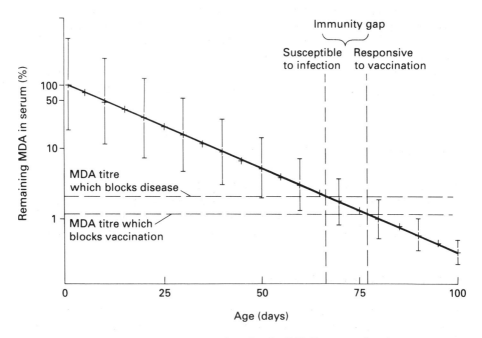

Figure 1 Effect of maternally derived antibody (MDA) on vaccination

- Extra doses of vaccine earlier and/or later than standard may be given. For example, earlier doses may be given during an outbreak of disease or when puppies or kittens are deprived of colostrum and are known to be at risk. Later doses might be appropriate if the mother is likely to pass on high levels of MDA, for example if there was a history of clinical disease.

Figure 1 shows the decline in serum levels of maternally derived antibody (MDA) in puppies and kittens. Approximately 80–98% MDA in puppies and kittens is derived from colostrum, that is from milk absorbed during the first 24 hours after birth. The graph demonstrates the decline in antibody titre (half-life approximated at 10 days) over the first 100 days of life, and the dotted lines indicate how variation in initial titre between and within litters can affect how long MDA persists. This shows how vaccines given too early will be blocked by MDA, and that, because attenuated vaccine viruses are less virulent than wild-type viruses, there will almost always be a short period (the immunity gap) when effective vaccination is impossible but the animal is susceptible to wild-type infection and disease. Furthermore, through variation in antibody titre in queens and bitches and in colostrum uptake by puppies and kittens, the optimum vaccination time will differ between individuals.

Vaccination of adult cats and dogs

- For many vaccines, only one dose is necessary to provide protection in an animal over 12 weeks old.
- Annual revaccination is recommended for most vaccines, although some (for example distemper) may need only be given every other year, while more frequent dosing may be advised for others (for example the intranasal *Bordetella bronchiseptica* kennel cough vaccine).
- The first booster at one year of age is, however, important in case the first vaccination course was for some reason ineffective, e.g. if MDA was still at interfering levels.

APPARENT VACCINE REACTIONS

Here the disease appears to be caused by the vaccine. Apparent reactions usually occur within a week or so of vaccination. True reactions may be due to either the biological component (i.e. the virus or bacterium) or some other component of the vaccine (usually the adjuvant), but many apparent reactions have other causes.

Apparent biological reactions

- Incomplete attenuation of virus or bacterial component. This is uncommon but not unknown, which is why suspected reactions should always be reported to the manufacturer and/or other appropriate bodies.

- Animal particularly susceptible to infection with attenuated pathogen. For example, a live vaccine given to a very young puppy or kitten or an immunosuppressed individual (e.g. owing to pre-existing infection with an immunosuppressive agent such as feline leukaemia virus, distemper or a parvovirus).
- Vaccine given by incorrect route. For example, live cat 'flu vaccines attenuated for subcutaneous injection will often cause disease if given oronasally (e.g. if cat licks vaccine left at injection site or inhales aerosol made when filling syringe).
- Animal infected and incubating disease at time of vaccination. As can be seen in Figure 1, puppies and kittens are often vaccinated just when maternal antibody levels are declining and so the animal is most susceptible to infection. This is probably the single most common reason for apparent biological reactions to vaccination at 8 or 9 weeks old.
- Animal a carrier of clinically inapparent infection. The stress of vaccination may induce shedding with some clinical signs in, for example, cats latently infected with felid herpesvirus-1.
- It is normal for some live vaccines to provoke mild clinical signs. Subcutaneous injection of many live vaccines gives rise to mild systemic clinical signs such as depression, lethargy and inappetance, generally lasting only 24 hours. Intranasal vaccines often cause mild signs of upper respiratory tract disease including sneezing and, sometimes, limited ocular or nasal discharges.

Apparent reactions to non-biological components of the vaccine

These are usually due to an inappropriate response to the adjuvant or a particular adjuvant–antigen combination.

- Mild skin reactions at the site of subcutaneous injection. Subcutaneous injection sometimes causes a mild local inflammatory response which may develop into a longer lasting granulomatous lesion. Such reactions generally cause the animal little discomfort, but in some breeds of cats may cause a change in colour of new hair growth. For this reason it may be advisable to use an injection site in such cats where any change in hair colour will be less obvious than the scruff (for example on the chest where hidden by a fore-limb).
- Sarcoma formation at the site of subcutaneous injection. Sarcoma formation at the site of injection has been associated with some vaccines using aluminium-based adjuvants in cats. In one survey, most were fibrosarcomas or malignant fibrous histiocytomas, although some osteosarcomas, rhabdomyosarcomas and chondrosarcomas were also reported. The authors of the survey suggested that rabies vaccines might be particularly implicated.
- Generalised mild reactions. Occasionally transient depression and pyrexia may be seen after vaccination, the underlying mechanism for which is unclear.

- Generalised hypersensitivity reactions
  - ○ Acute anaphylactic reactions can occur with the use of any vaccine, but are particularly associated with the use of killed adjuvanted vaccines. In both cats and dogs, the signs are of vomiting and diarrhoea within minutes or hours of vaccination and severe respiratory distress (dyspnoea and cyanosis). Adrenaline or corticosteroids should be given promptly.
  - ○ Autoimmune anaemias occurring within a few weeks of vaccination have also been reported in both cats and dogs.

APPARENT VACCINE BREAKDOWNS

Here there is development of the disease despite vaccination. Apparent breakdowns usually occur several weeks or more after vaccination but within the normal described period of immunity. Possible causes of apparent vaccine breakdown include:

- Faulty (non-potent) vaccine. Uncommon, but possible. Report suspected cases to the manufacturer and/or other appropriate body.
- Incorrect storage of vaccine. A likely cause of non-potency. Do not use vaccines after their recommended use-by date, and always store them according to the manufacturer's instructions. Live vaccines are particularly liable to lose potency if stored incorrectly.
- Incorrect administration of vaccine. Most frequently the result of the injection of an inadequate dose of vaccine (for example through the skin twice). Administration by the wrong route (for example intranasal vaccines given subcutaneously or killed systemic vaccines given oronasally) will also be ineffective at provoking protective immunity.
- Inhibition of vaccination by maternally derived antibody. A common cause of apparent vaccine failure in young animals. If the last vaccine dose is given before the puppy or kitten is 12 weeks old, or if the animal has particularly high MDA, vaccination may not provide active immunity and protection.
- Animal already infected. Vaccination rarely prevents the development of disease in an already infected animal or elimination of a carrier state. Vaccination of carriers of viruses such as feline calicivirus and felid herpesvirus-1, which can cause persistent infection, will not provoke elimination of infection and these animals may later shed virus and sometimes develop clinical disease.
- Intercurrent disease or immunosuppression. Infection with immunosuppressive agents, either at the time of vaccination or later, may prevent or decrease protective vaccine-derived immunity.
- Infection with different organisms or strains from those contained in the vaccine. Before a clinical disease can be ascribed to vaccine breakdown, the causative organism(s) must be identified. Cat 'flu and kennel cough, for example, are clinical descriptions of syndromes with multifactorial aetiology, and some causes of infectious upper respiratory disease in cats and dogs are

not included in any vaccine. Similarly, not all cases of haemorrhagic gastro-enteritis in dogs are caused by canine parvovirus.

- Overwhelming infection. Vaccines generally provide reasonable protection against the development of disease, but not against infection. Thus, infection with very large doses of a pathogen, particularly if vaccine derived immunity is beginning to wane, will sometimes lead to clinical disease.

FURTHER READING

This section is not meant to be an exhaustive reference source. The reader is mainly referred to the textbooks listed below for reviews of established infectious diseases (e.g. feline panleucopenia). A further selection of recent and topical references is given under the individual section headings including vaccination.

GENERAL TEXTS

Appel, M.J. (1987) *Virus Infections of Carnivores*. Elsevier Science BV, Amsterdam, The Netherlands.
August, J.R. (1994) *Consultations in Feline Internal Medicine 2*. W.B. Saunders Company, London.
Chandler, E.A., Gaskell, C.J. & Gaskell, R.M. (1994) *Feline Medicine and Therapeutics*, 2nd Edn. Blackwell Science, Oxford.
Ettinger, S.J. & Feldman, E.C. (1995) *Textbook of Veterinary Internal Medicine*. W.B. Saunders Company, London.
Greene, C.E. (1990) *Infectious Diseases of the Dog and Cat*. W.B. Saunders Company, London.
Gorman, N. (1996) *Canine Medicine and Therapeutics*, 4th edn. Blackwell Science, Oxford.
Sherding, R.G. (1994) *The Cat: Diseases and Clinical Management*, 2nd edn, Vol. 1. Churchill Livingstone, Edinburgh.
Tennant, B. (1994) *Small Animal Formulary*. British Small Animal Veterinary Association Publications, Cheltenham.

MAJOR FELINE INFECTIOUS DISEASES

Addie, D.D. *et al.* (1995) Risk of feline infectious peritonitis in cats naturally infected with feline coronavirus. *American Journal of Veterinary Research* **56**, 429.
Bennett, M. & Baxby, D. (1995) Feline and human cowpox. In: *Veterinary Annual*, (eds M.-E. Raw & T.J. Parkinson), 35th edn. Blackwell Science, Oxford.
Brown, E.W. *et al.* (1994) A lion lentivirus related to feline immunodeficiency virus – epidemiologic and phylogenetic aspects. *Journal of Virology* **68**, 5953.
English, R.V. *et al.* (1994) Development of clinical disease in cats experimentally infected with feline immunodeficiency virus. *Journal of Infectious Diseases* **170**, 543.

Gruffydd-Jones, T.J. *et al.* (1992) Feline spongiform encephalopathy. *Journal of Small Animal Practice* **33**, 471.

Gunn-Moore, D.A. *et al.* (1995) Prevalence of *Chlamydia psittaci* antibodies in healthy pet cats in Britain. *Veterinary Record* **136**, 366.

Herrewegh, A.A.P.M. *et al.* (1995) Detection of feline coronavirus RNA in faeces, tissues and body fluids of naturally-infected cats by reverse-transcriptase PCR. *Journal of Clinical Microbiology* **33**, 684.

Jacobs, A.A.C. *et al.* (1993) Feline bordetellosis: challenge and vaccine studies. *Veterinary Record* **133**, 260.

Jarrett, O. *et al.* (1991) Comparison of diagnostic methods for feline leukaemia virus and feline immunodeficiency virus. *Journal of the American Veterinary Medical Association* **199**, 1362.

McArdle, H.C. *et al.* Seroprevalence and isolation rate of *Bordetella bronchiseptica* in cats in the UK. *Veterinary Record* **135**, 506.

Nasisse, M.P. *et al.* (1993) Clinical and laboratory findings in chronic conjunctivitis in cats – 91 cases (1983–91). *Journal of the American Veterinary Medical Association* **203**, 834.

Pedersen, N.C. (1995) An overview of feline enteric coronavirus and infectious peritonitis virus infections. *Feline Practice* **23** (3), 7.

Pedersen, N.C., Addie, D. & Wolf, A. (1995) Recommendations from working groups of the international feline enteric coronavirus and feline infectious peritonitis workshop. *Feline Practice* **23** (3), 108.

Reubel, G.H., Hoffmann, D.E. & Pedersen, N.C. (1992) Acute and chronic faucitis of domestic cats. A feline calicivirus-induced disease. *Veterinary Clinics of North America – Small Animal Practice* **22**, 1347.

Squires, R.A. & Gorman, N.T. (1990) Anti-neoplastic chemotherapy in cats. *In Practice* **12**, 101.

Swenson, C.L. *et al.* (1993) Eosinophilic leukemia in a cat with naturally acquired feline leukemia virus infection. *Journal of the American Animal Hospital Association* **29**, 497.

MAJOR CANINE INFECTIOUS DISEASES

Bell, S.C. *et al.* (1991) Canine distemper viral antigens and antibodies in dogs with rheumatoid arthritis. *Research in Veterinary Science* **50**, 64.

Bemis, D.A. (1992) *Bordetella* and *Mycoplasma* respiratory infections in dogs and cats. *Veterinary Clinics of North America – Small Animal Practice* **22**, 1173.

Beynon, P.H. & Edney, A.T.B. (Eds) *Rabies in a Changing World.* Symposium, Royal Society of Medicine, British Small Animal Veterinary Association, Royal Society of Health, London, May 1995.

Blixenkronemoller, M. *et al.* (1993) Studies on manifestations of canine distemper virus infection in an urban dog population. *Veterinary Microbiology* **37**, 163.

Gordon, M.T., Anderson, D.C. & Sharpe, P.T. (1991) Canine distemper virus localised in bone-cells of patients with Paget's disease. *Bone* **12**, 195.

Gordon, M.T. *et al.* (1993) Prevalence of canine distemper antibodies in the pagetic population. *Journal of Medical Microbiology* **40**, 313.

Johnson, C.A. & Walker, R.D. (1992) Clinical signs and diagnosis of *Brucella canis* infection. *Compendium on Continuing Education for the Practicing Veterinarian* **14**, 763.

Mee, A.P. *et al.* (1992) Detection of canine distemper virus in bone cells in the metaphyses of distemper-infected dogs. *Journal of Bone and Mineral Research* **7**, 829.

Parrish, C.R. *et al.* (1991) Rapid antigenic-type replacement and DNA sequence evolution of canine parvovirus. *Journal of Urology* **65**, 6544.

Pastoret, P.-P., Boulanger, D. & Brochier, B. (1995) The rabies situation in Europe. In: *The Veterinary Annual*, (eds M.-E. Raw & T.J. Parkinson), 35th edn. Blackwell Science, Oxford.

Raw, M.-E. *et al.* (1992) Canine distemper infection associated with acute nervous signs in dogs. *Veterinary Record* **130**, 291.

Tennant, B.J. *et al.* (1991) Prevalence of antibodies to four major canine viral diseases in dogs in a Liverpool hospital population. *Journal of Small Animal Practice* **32**, 175.

Tennant, B.J. *et al.* (1993) Studies on the epizootiology of canine coronavirus. *Veterinary Record* **132**, 7.

Tipold, A., Vandevelde, M. & Jaggy, A. (1992) Neurological manifestations of canine distemper virus infection. *Journal of Small Animal Practice* **33**, 466.

MISCELLANEOUS VIRAL INFECTIONS

Bennett, M. *et al.* (1990) The prevalence of antibody to *Hantavirus* in some cat populations in Britain. *Veterinary Record* **127**, 548.

Lundgren, A.-L. (1992) Feline non-suppurative meningoencephalomyelitis. A clinical and pathological study. *Journal of Comparative Pathology* **107**, 411.

Modiano, J.F. *et al.* (1995) Retrovirus-like activity in an immunosuppressed dog – pathological and immunological findings. *Journal of Comparative Pathology* **112**, 165.

Muir, P. *et al.* (1990) A clinical and microbiological study of cats with nictitating membrane protrusion and diarrhoea; isolation of a novel virus. *Veterinary Record* **127**, 324.

Nowotny, N. & Weissenbröck, H. (1995) Description of feline nonsuppurative meningoencephalomyelitis ('staggering disease') and studies of its etiology. *Journal of Clinical Microbiology* **33**, 1668.

MISCELLANEOUS BACTERIAL INFECTIONS

Allaker, R.P., Langlois, T. and Hardie, J.M. (1994) Prevalence of *Eikenella corrodens* and *Actinobacillus actinomycetem comitans* in dental plaque of dogs. *Veterinary Record* **134**, 519.

Chomel, B.B. *et al.* (1994) Serological surveillance of plague in dogs and cats, California, 1979–1991. *Comparative Immunology, Microbiology and Infectious Diseases* **17**, 111.

Corboz, L., Ossent, P. & Gruber, H. (1993) Lokale und sytemische Infektionen mit Bakterien der Gruppe EF-4 bei Hunden, Katzen und bei einem Dachs: Bakteriologische und Pathologisch-anatomische Befunde. *Schweizer Archiv für Tierheilkunde* **135**, 96.

Eidson, M., Thilsted, J.P. & Rollag, O.J. (1991) Clinical, clinipathologic and pathological features of plague in cats: 119 cases (1977–88). *Journal of the American Veterinary Medical Association* **119**, 1191.

Fox, J.G. *et al.* (1995) *Helicobacter pylori*-induced gastritis in the domestic cat. *Infection and Immunity* **63**, 2674.

Koehler, J.E., Glaser, C.A. & Tappero, J.W. (1994) *Rochalimaea henselae* infection: a new zoonosis with the domestic cat as reservoir. *Journal of the American Medical Association* **271**, 531.

Jordan, H.L., Cohn, L.A. & Armstrong, P.J. (1994) Disseminated *Mycobacterium avium* complex infection in three Siamese cats. *Journal of the American Veterinary Medical Association* **204**, 90.

FUNGAL, ALGAL AND PROTOZOAL INFECTIONS

Dubey, J.P. & Carpenter, J.L. (1993) Neonatal toxoplasmosis in littermate cats. *Journal of the American Veterinary Medical Association* **203**, 1546.

Dubey, J.P. & Carpenter, J.L. (1993) Histologically confirmed clinical toxoplasmosis in cats – 100 cases (1952-1990). *Journal of the American Veterinary Medical Association* **203**, 1556.

Greene, R.T. & Troy, G.C. (1995) Coccidiomycosis in 48 cats – a retrospective study (1984-1993). *Journal of Veterinary Internal Medicine* **9**, 86.

Mtambo, M.M. *et al.* (1991) *Cryptosporidium* infection in cats: prevalence of infection in domestic and feral cats in the Glasgow area. *Veterinary Record* **129**, 502.

Sato, K., Iwamoto, I. & Yoshiki, K. (1993) Experimental toxoplasmosis in pregnant cats. *Journal of Veterinary Medicine and Science* **55**, 1005.

Werner, A.H. & Werner, B.E. (1993) Feline sporotrichosis. *Compendium on Continuing Education for the Practicing Veterinarian* **15**, 1189.

Wolf, A. (1992) Fungal diseases of the nasal cavity of the dog and cat. *Veterinary Clinics of North America – Small Animal Practice* **22**, 1119.

VACCINATION

Bell, J.A. *et al.* (1994) A formalin-inactivated vaccine protects against mucosal papillomavirus infection – a canine model. *Pathobiology* **62**, 194.

Chalmers, W.S.K. & Baxendale W. (1994) A comparison of canine distemper vaccine and measles vaccine for the prevention of canine distemper in young puppies. *Veterinary Record* **135**, 349.

Dawson, S. & Gaskell, R.M. (1993) Problems with respiratory virus vaccination in cats. *Compendium on Continuing Education for the Practicing Veterinarian* **15**, 1347.

Dawson, S. *et al.* (1993) Investigation of vaccine reactions and breakdowns after feline calicivirus vaccination. *Veterinary Record* **132**, 346.

Gerber, J.D. (1995) Overview of the development of a modified live temperature-sensitive FIP virus vaccine. *Feline Practice* **23** (3), 62.

Greenwood, N.M. *et al.* (1995) Comparison of isolates of canine parvovirus by restriction enzyme analysis, and vaccine efficacy against field strains. *Veterinary Record* **136**, 63.

Hendrick M.J. & Brooks J.J. (1994) Postvaccinal sarcomas in the cat: histology and immunohistology. *Veterinary Pathology* **31**, 126.

Hosie, M. (1994) The development of a vaccine against feline immunodeficiency virus. *British Veterinary Journal* **150**, 25.

Johnson CM *et al.* (1994) FIV as a model for AIDS vaccination. *AIDS Research and Human Retroviruses* **10**, 225.

Macy, D.W. (1994) Vaccination against feline retroviruses. *Consultations in Feline Internal Medicine 2*. W.B. Saunders Company, London, p.33.

INDEX

Page numbers in **bold** refer to the main discussions of the subject.